1000116337

D0530137

IMPLEMENTATION OF THE GLOBAL STRATEGY FOR HEALTH FOR ALL BY THE YEAR 2000

SECOND EVALUATION

EIGHTH REPORT ON THE WORLD HEALTH SITUATION

VOLUME 3
REGION OF THE AMERICAS

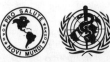

PAN AMERICAN HEALTH ORGANIZATION
Pan American Sanitary Bureau, Regional Office of the
WORLD HEALTH ORGANIZATION
525 Twenty-third Street, N.W.
Washington, D.C. 20037, USA
1993

1 00 011633 7

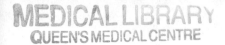
MEDICAL LIBRARY
QUEEN'S MEDICAL CENTRE

Spanish edition (1993):
Aplicación de la Estrategia Mundial de Salud para Todos en el Año 2000
ISBN 92 4 360283 7 (OMS)
ISBN 92 75 37250 0 (OPS)

French edition (1993):
Mise en oeuvre de la stratégie mondiale de la santé pour tous d'ici l'an 2000
ISBN 92 4 260283 3 (OMS)
ISBN 92 75 07250 7 (OPS)

PAHO Library Cataloguing in Publication Data

Pan American Health Organization
   Implementation of the global strategy for Health for All by the Year 2000 :
second evaluation : eighth report on the world health situation : vol. 3, region of
the Americas.
   Washington, D.C. : PAHO, © 1993. — vi, 126 p.

   ISBN 92 75 17250 1

I. Title   1. HEALTH FOR ALL BY THE YEAR 2000
2. WORLD STRATEGIES   3. AMERICA
4. EVALUATION OF PUBLIC HEALTH INTERVENTIONS (PROCESS
   AND OUTCOME)   5. PAHO
NLM: WA540.1

924160283X

ISBN 92 4 160283 X (WHO)
ISBN 92 75 17250 1 (PAHO)

The Pan American Health Organization welcomes requests for permission to reproduce or translate its publications, in part or in full. Applications and inquiries should be addressed to the Publications Program, Pan American Health Organization, 525 23rd St., N.W., Washington, D.C., 20037, U.S.A., which will be glad to provide the latest information on any changes made to the text, plans for new editions, and reprints and translations already available.

© Pan American Health Organization 1993

   Publications of the Pan American Health Organization enjoy copyright protection in accordance with the provisions of Protocol 2 of the Universal Copyright Convention. All rights are reserved.
   The designations employed and the presentation of the material in this publication do not imply the expression of any opinion whatsoever on the part of the Secretariat of the Pan American Health Organization concerning the status of any country, territory, city or area or of its authorities, or concerning the delimitation of its frontiers or boundaries.
   The mention of specific companies or of certain manufacturers' products does not imply that they are endorsed or recommended by the Pan American Health Organization in preference to others of a similar nature that are not mentioned. Errors and omissions excepted, the names of proprietary products are distinguished by initial capital letters.

PRINTED IN THE UNITED STATES OF AMERICA

CONTENTS

1000116337

Preface

This report covers the 1985–1990 period, and presents the results and level attained by the countries of the Americas in their efforts to arrive at the goal of health for all by the year 2000.

The economic, political, and social difficulties that most of the countries have experienced during this period have to some extent influenced the level of progress toward the goal of health for all by the year 2000. The health services' coverage and quality problems, the reliance on technologically complex curative care, excessive centralization, the sector's financing problems, and the community's restricted participation in health services planning and administration are still prevalent in many countries, and in recent years, these problems have deepened in several of the countries. The rise in relative and absolute poverty that has taken place in recent years, has increased the marginalization of vast segments of the population from access to all services, and to the health services in particular—all of which has amplified existing inequalities and inequities.

The resolutions that the countries adopted in Alma-Ata endorsed the notion that health is linked to the population's living conditions, and that it should not be viewed merely as the absence of disease; that in order to care for health, comprehensive social responses are needed that allow each individual and the entire population to benefit from health promotion, preservation, and recovery activities.

If the goal of health for all is to be attained, the Region's countries and the Organization still have a long road to travel in the short time before the end of the century.

Nowadays, continually monitoring and periodically evaluating the health conditions of different social groups have become more important for guiding high-level political decisions that seek efficient and equitable social interventions. The economic transformation and adjustment policies that the countries pursue as they attempt to once again experience growth and development, must consider, as their highest priority, their effect on the living conditions, the health, and the welfare of the populations. By the same token, the health sector's transformation processes must take into consideration their impact on the economy and political stability.

Making health one of the inherent elements of development while simultaneously reshaping the organization and guidelines of the heath sector, is the great challenge that we face in the near future as citizens, professionals, and public health institutions.

CARLYLE GUERRA DE MACEDO
DIRECTOR
PAN AMERICAN SANITARY BUREAU
REGIONAL OFFICE OF THE
WORLD HEALTH ORGANIZATION
FOR THE AMERICAS

Introduction

The Member States of WHO unanimously adopted the Global Strategy for Health for All by the Year 2000 in 1977 (Resolution WHA30.43), and, subsequently, the Plan of Action for its implementation. They also agreed to monitor progress in the implementation of their national strategies and to evaluate at regular intervals their effectiveness in improving the health status of the population. The World Health Assembly proposed that the corresponding reports be analyzed every two years by the regional committees, the Executive Board, and the World Health Assembly, and that every six years an evaluation be performed to determine the effectiveness and impact of the strategy on national, regional, and global plans. The process was initiated in 1983 with a first monitoring report, which was followed in 1985 by a first evaluation of the effectiveness of the implementation of national strategies, and in 1988 by a second monitoring report. The 39th World Health Assembly (Resolution WHA39.7) decided to institute the submission of monitoring reports on the strategy every six years, beginning in 1985.

To facilitate the presentation of systematic reports and the summary of information at the regional and world levels, a common framework of reference was adopted. In 1982, a Common Framework and Format (CFF) was prepared by WHO to aid in the collection and analysis of the information needed in order to monitor progress in the implementation of the national strategies and report it to the regional committees, the Executive Board, and the World Health Assembly. Subsequently, an expanded CFF was prepared for reporting on the evaluation of the effectiveness of the strategies' implementation. The Common Framework: Second Evaluation (CFE/2), which was utilized in preparing the present evaluation, is the result of modifications to the CFF made as a result of observations and suggestions from the Member States and Regional Offices.

On the basis of the experience acquired during the evaluation carried out in this Region during 1984–1985 and during the monitoring process in 1988, the decision was made to send the CFE/2 to the countries to guide them in the preparation of their national reports. In addition, the PAHO/WHO Country Representatives were urged to provide all necessary support and collaboration to enable every country to measure its progress, discover any problems, locate obstacles, and, ultimately, utilize the results of the analysis to improve its health plans.

A total of 28 countries and territories submitted reports: Argentina, Bahamas, Belize, Bolivia, Brazil, Canada, Chile, Colombia, Costa Rica, Cuba, the Dominican Republic, Ecuador, El Salvador, Guatemala, Haiti, Guyana, Honduras, Jamaica, Mexico, Nicaragua, Panama, Paraguay, Peru, Suriname, Trinidad and Tobago, the United States of America, Uruguay, and Venezuela. Quantitative information also was received from Anguilla, Antigua, Barbados, the British Virgin Islands, Cayman Islands, Dominica, Grenada, Montserrat, Saint Kitts and Nevis, Saint Lucia, and Saint Vincent and the Grenadines. These countries and political units represent almost 100% of the population in the Region of the Americas. The analysis of specific indicators took into account not only the national reports received, but also complementary sources (World Bank, IDB, UNESCO, UNICEF, UNDP, ECLAC, United Nations Statistical Office, IMF) and information from PAHO technical areas and previous reports from the countries to PAHO.

The consolidated regional report covers the following subjects: socioeconomic status, monitoring process and mechanisms, national health policies and strategies, development of health sys-

1

tems, international action, availability of primary health care, and health status and living conditions. This analysis of the evaluation of the strategies of health for all by the year 2000 is based on the information submitted in accordance with the Common Framework: Second Evaluation; consequently, it includes only the answers of the 28 countries which followed the CFE/2 format in their reports. On the other hand, the tables (see Annex) include all the countries and political units which submitted quantitative data.

REGIONAL EVALUATION

Chapter 1

Socioeconomic status

In terms of their economies, the countries of Latin America and the Caribbean ended the 1980s and began the 1990s (1988, 1989, and 1990) immersed in a prolonged recession, carrying large external debt liabilities and confronting a basic maladjustment in the structures of international demand and the makeup of exports. These economic setbacks, which had strong social consequences, led some to call the 1980s the "lost decade," reflecting the magnitude of the crisis in the Region during that period.

One of the global indicators—the per capita gross domestic product (GDP)—declined for the third consecutive year in 1990, decreasing by 2.6% (it had decreased 0.6% in 1989 and 1.2% in 1988), which constituted a cumulative change of −9.6% for the period 1981–1990. Several difficulties remain, including macroeconomic imbalances, obsolescence of the capital and physical plant infrastructure, a widening gap between worldwide technological changes and those that are occurring in the Region, misuse of the financial and managerial capacity of the governments, growing frustration on the part of those trying to enter the job market (especially in urban areas), growing inflation in an increasing number of countries, and poor utilization of natural resources with the ensuing damage to the environment.

In the course of the decade, the deterioration in trade terms, the external debt service, and decreased foreign capital income reduced the net resources available for investment. The net investment ratio for the Region fell from almost 23% in 1980 to 16.5% in 1988. This had far-reaching implications for central government expenditure as a percentage of GDP, because a large increase in the amount allocated for debt payment is coupled with a reduction in capital outlay. According to ECLAC, the 1980s crisis in the countries of Latin America and the Caribbean was characterized by a loss of dynamism in national economies, intractable macroeconomic imbalances, the regressive nature of the adjustment and social deterioration, weakening of the public sector, and a marked decline in investments.

The net transfer of resources to other countries, which had already been negative over the three-year period from 1985 to 1987 (24 billion dollars annually), continues to drain Latin America and the Caribbean. It amounted to 25 billion annually over the three-year period between 1988 and 1990. The balance of trade continues to be positive (basically due to the increase in exports), totaling 27 billion annually during 1988–1990; it has been used to pay the debt, or rather the debt's interest, since the total gross external debt has remained constant at 420 billion over 1987–1990. Given this stagnation in production and the Region's characteristics, which basically involve exporting raw materials, the foregoing figures imply a reduced availability of essential products for domestic consumption.

The impact of increased unemployment, the government's lowered social expenditure, and decreased availability of products for domestic consumption is evident when the extent of the poverty in Latin America in the 1980s is analyzed. By the end of 1980, 37% of families were considered poor and 17%, indigent. Estimates for 1989 indicate that there are some 183 million people living in poverty (44% of the total population). This figure is 71 million more than in 1970. Of the 1989 total, 88 million people were classified as indigent (21% of the total population), 28 million more than in 1970. This growing impoverishment has been particularly marked in urban areas.

During the late 1980s, supposedly sweeping reform programs were developed in most of the Latin American and Caribbean countries. Some were tentative and others superficial, some were successful and others were not. Despite their differences, all these programs shared one characteristic: an acknowledgment of the importance of international trade and public financing in promoting growth and consumption, although the instability of international markets and the protectionist policies of many developed countries (in this regard, the failure of the GATT round is very clear) have hindered the entry of the Region's products into international markets. Recent events point to an increase in trade between subregions; treaties have already been signed in North America (Canada and the United States of America) and in South America (Argentina, Brazil, Paraguay, Uruguay); others are under study (Central America; the Andean countries; and Canada, the United States of America, and Mexico).

Although the 1980s were marked by economic and social setbacks, the decade witnessed some notable political advances. By the mid-1980s, several democracies had already been strengthened, and the trend was further accentuated when democracy returned to Chile, Haiti, and Paraguay between 1988 and 1990, although the events in Panama interrupted this process. In other words, in the 1980s, especially in the decade's later years, there was a concurrence of trends in the Region. Political dialogue was strengthened, but at the same time public institutions were debilitated. Economic regression coexisted with structural reform programs that have yet to produce desired results. Exports increased, but at the expense of investment and consumption. And the social costs were high: increases in unemployment and poverty and decreases in the quality of education and health services coincided with the development of social emergency programs for the neediest groups, the impact of which has been difficult to evaluate given the lack of focus and clarity regarding their functions.

In its analysis, ECLAC states that Latin America and the Caribbean are presently at a crossroads, and that they must find their way back to the road that leads to development, from which they seem to have strayed in the turbulence of the past decade. Overcoming the crisis will necessitate an extraordinary accumulation of needs. For example, there is, on the one hand, a need to strengthen democracy; on the other, economies must be adjusted, stabilized, and incorporated into the fast-paced process of worldwide technological change, and public sectors must be modernized, savings increased, income distribution improved, and more austere patterns of consumption implemented. And all of this must be done in the context of a sustained development.

Another consideration, although not one of the indicators, is the cholera epidemic, which in early 1991 reappeared, for the first time this century, in several Latin American countries with varying degrees of socioeconomic and sanitary development. The epidemic revealed all too clearly the profound deficiencies that persist in the Region's countries.

Chapter 2

Monitoring and evaluation process and mechanisms

The efforts to promote the processes of monitoring and evaluation at various levels of the sector, as described in the 1988 monitoring report, have weakened. No country in Latin America has reported the existence of (or attempts to create) a specialized unit for the monitoring and evaluation of health for all by the year 2000 and primary health care. Since 1988, only two countries in the Region have reported having defined their goals and objectives with regard to health for all by the year 2000. In the document "Health for All: A Framework for Health Promotion," Canada has clearly outlined its goals and objectives regarding health for all by the year 2000, including reducing inequities, enhancing coping, and building supportive environments. In the United States of America, the document "Healthy People 2000" was prepared in 1990, following an evaluation of the goals established in 1980 and through a broad participatory process (involving more than 800 organizations in two years). Perhaps the most widely seen feature in the countries reporting from Latin America is the near total absence of any attempt at evaluating the previously proposed targets and goals, regardless of whether or not they fell within the framework of health for all by the year 2000 and primary health care. Another important consideration is the failure to establish national (and regional) indicators for specific problems in every country from the outset of the process of development and commitment that began with the Declaration of Alma Ata. As is stated in the report of El Salvador: "There is no true process of identification and updating of the indicators necessary for planning, monitoring, and evaluation." And as long as there is no real evaluation, the process of collecting and using information will be intrinsically weak.

The availability of data for the different indicators varies considerably. The registries from which information is obtained for the calculations of various indicators related to natality (specific rates, fertility, general fertility, gross rates) and mortality (specific rates, life tables, cause of death) hardly exist in two of the reporting countries—Bolivia and Haiti—and data from them cannot be used. There are several countries with varying degrees of underregistration, both between countries and within the same country, and data from them therefore may not be entirely reliable: Brazil, Colombia, the Dominican Republic, Ecuador, El Salvador, Guatemala, Guyana, Honduras, Mexico, Nicaragua, Paraguay, Peru, Suriname, and Venezuela (the last being on the borderline with the previous group). Finally, there are countries whose registration system is complete (or nearly complete) and the data from them can be used to calculate rates: Argentina, Bahamas, Belize, Canada, Chile, Costa Rica, Cuba, Jamaica, Panama, the United States, and Uruguay. Moreover, in recent years, some countries have launched efforts to prevent the deterioration of their vital statistics systems and to hold on to previous advances in this regard (Argentina, for example). This has meant that in many countries the most important indicators come from estimates derived from censuses or special surveys.

Immunization remains the area for which the most timely information is available (both at the country and regional levels) in terms of coverage, with all the countries reporting on immunization in their national reports. Next is basic sanitation, although in many cases the data are not broken down into urban and rural components. In this area there is a definite need for continuous updating and perhaps for more precision, since many data are not comparable. The United States reports on drinking water and excreta disposal services in households with connections, and, therefore, its data are lower than those of other countries that report on population with "reasonable or easy access." There continue to be problems regarding the data on maternal and child health services: birthweight is reported in 19 countries; weight-for-height (or similar) indicators, in 8 countries; proportion of pregnant women immunized against tetanus, in 16; and attended pregnancies in 19. Furthermore, many of these indicators do not come from ongoing registry systems that provide total coverage and break down the data in such a way as to make them useful for programming activities. The primary health care coverage indicator continues to be difficult to estimate because not all the countries are capable of calculating it, and some figures are inconsistent with other indicators. Thus, a country may show a high (94%) rate of primary health care coverage, and yet the individual figures for the primary health care component indicators are much lower. There has been little understanding of the new indicator of probability of dying before the age of 5 years. Few countries have calculated it at all, and of those that have, some have figured it as a rate and not as a probability. The maternal mortality indicator has shown the most improvement because comparatively more figures are presented (21) and it also corresponds to the years following the monitoring report.

The reliability of data comparisons on percentage of GNP spent on health is questionable, since some reports only deal with the central government, and others include smaller political and administrative units; some take into account social security expenditure and others do not. Argentina reports data from surveys that also include private out-of-pocket expenditures. Furthermore, there is no uniformity regarding the amounts allocated for public health care, and most of the countries report that they are unable to make these calculations. The area of financing and expenditure in Latin America and the Caribbean is a great void. Data on literacy basically come from population censuses that are conducted every 10 years, usually at the beginning of each decade; data for the periods between censuses are estimated. Owing to problems associated with the lack of comparability (differences in year, currency, trends, constants, etc.), this report does not include data from the countries concerning GNP or GDP (global and/or per capita). These data have been taken from other sources.

Data regarding human resources were received from 19 countries, although some only report on the public sector. Thirteen countries reported total beds in the country, four reported only those corresponding to the public sector (MPH, SS, or both), and ten did not report.

With respect to mortality by cause, only five countries did not report; of these, information is available for two (Chile and Guatemala). Some of the countries reported only the order of the main causes. With regard to morbidity, there are 12 countries that did not report at all; for the other 15, the data are not readily comparable, both because of underregistration and because they refer to different aspects of morbidity (discharges, outpatient consultation, required reporting). For both morbidity and mortality, each case must be studied individually in order to assess the usefulness of the reported data.

One particular phenomenon should be pointed out—the national reports generally contain less information than exists and is available in the countries themselves. Sometimes data are received for a certain year and more current data actually exist; other times no data are sent, when they could be found if a true process of investigation were undertaken. This applies especially to the information on services, since the information sent tends to concern the public sector, overlooking not only the private sector but social security as well. In this regard, there have been noteworthy advances in Mexico, with the establishment of the National Health Information System (SNIS), which includes social security institutions, and in Costa Rica, with the legal establishment of the National Health System.

Several obstacles hinder monitoring and surveillance, but they all basically stem from the low priority that has been assigned to health for all by the year 2000 and primary health care in recent years. Decision-making has been dominated by political and economic considerations (changes in political authorities, economic restrictions), which has led to a limited utilization of the data generated (whether the amount was large or small), lack of coordination, and institutional breakup. It is not surprising that there continue to be problems derived from the scarcity of human resources (quantity, quality, distribution) and large gaps in data: underregistration, scattered sources, untimely delivery, insufficient use of local level resources, and lack of conceptual uniformity within the different levels and services.

The main steps that are being taken in the countries to strengthen the evaluation of health for all are indirect, since they do not derive from a plan of priorities established specifically to that end, but rather come out of attempts to rationalize the use of limited resources. Among the most noteworthy of these steps are decentralization and the introduction of computerized systems. But much work remains to be done in order to ensure the availability of complete, timely, and comparable information for evaluation and monitoring.

Chapter 3

National health policies and strategies

In recent years various plans, policies, and strategies have been formulated, and all of them have components directly related to health for all by the year 2000 and primary health care and are in accord with them. Notable among them because of the emphasis being placed on them in the countries, and consistent with the trend observed three years ago, are decentralization, being implemented through different approaches, and the development of local health systems.

Efforts to strengthen national health systems are illustrated by several plans:

Belize: The National Health Plan 1990, which has been conceived on the basis of democratic, comprehensive, educational, and participatory principles, proposes accessibility to services, health promotion, intersectoral coordination, and community involvement as components.

Bolivia: The National Plan of Survival, Child Development and Maternal Health (1989) was characterized by a policy of decentralization and community involvement.

Canada: Following the plan for Achieving Health for All in 1986, several important programs have been developed, including Mental Health for Canadians and Drug Strategy. The Health and Environment Action Plan is currently being developed.

Colombia: The process of decentralization begun in 1986 was formalized with the passage in 1990 of Law 10 (Restructuring of the National Health System). A product of this law was the development of the Quadrennial Plan 1991–1994: Health with Democracy—Healthy Families in a Healthy Environment.

Costa Rica: Previous policies, especially those related to coordinating the activities of public health and social security, led to the legal adoption of the National Regulations for the National Health System (Executive Decree of November 1989). National health policy and strategy priorities are: promotion, care for special groups, environmental health, local health systems, human resources, infrastructure, and development of the national health service.

Ecuador: The National Health Plan 1989–1992 has the following priorities—integral family and community health, food and nutrition, basic sanitation, drugs, and hospital care.

El Salvador: The National Health Plan 1991–1994 (framed within the Economic and Social Development Plan) emphasizes focused expenditure and food aid and modernization of the administration of services and food aid.

Honduras: Based on two documents, "Leadership and Management of the Ministry of Public Health in 1990–1994" and "Global Response of the Ministry of Public Health to the Effects of Structural Adjustment in the Honduran Economy," a plan of action was developed that included effectiveness and efficiency in services; immunization; drugs; environment, nutrition, and health; and monitoring of living conditions among deprived groups.

Mexico: As part of the National Development Plan 1989–1994, the National Health Plan 1990–1994 was formulated (January 1991), which established promotion of a culture of health, universal access with equity and quality, prevention and control of disease and accidents, protection of the environment and basic sanitation, regulation of population growth, and promotion of social welfare as political guidelines.

Paraguay: The Plan for Immediate Actions in Health (1989) established the bases for the current Strategic Sectoral Health Plan. This is complemented by the National Plan for the Second Drinking Water Decade and the National Program for Human Development, which is addressed to the population living in dire poverty.

United States of America: The program Healthy People 2000: National Health Promotion and Disease Prevention Objectives (1990) encompasses three major goals—to increase the number of healthy years of life, to reduce inequities in health status among population groups, and to provide access to preventive services for the entire population. Twenty-two priority areas were defined with 300 quantified objectives.

In Chile, as a result of the major political changes that occurred in 1990, a review of policies and strategies is being conducted with a view to preparing new future goals and objectives. The same process is being carried out in Panama. In Argentina, under Law 23661 on the National Health Insurance System, which passed in December 1988, efforts are being made to regulate, coordinate, and extend coverage to the indigent, and this is being carried out within a process of state reform, decentralization, and privatization. In Brazil, the Constitution of 1988 formalizes the strategic principles of primary health care, creating the Unified Health System that integrates public health and social security and, as a clear move toward decentralization, transfers health care units to the states and *municipios*. Cuba, with a high level system of services, has set the following priorities: prevention and promotion through the family doctor; development of a network of specialties; training, specialization, and continuing education for human resources; and scientific research on the pharmaceutical industry and production of medical equipment. In Haiti, a coordination unit for the Health Priority Program was created, and seven priorities were established: diarrheal diseases and maternal nutrition, immunization, maternal health and family planning, malnutrition, major endemic diseases, tuberculosis, and AIDS. In Peru, the Integrated National and Regional Health System was created with great emphasis on decentralization, and this occurred in the context of an unfavorable political and economic climate (Decree 351 of the Organic Law of the Health Sector was rescinded and the National Health Council is not functioning). In Suriname, the Regional Health Services have been taken out of the public sector and have become nongovernmental organizations (NGOs).

Obstacles to the implementation of national health policies and strategies vary, and in many cases are predictable. They include personnel restrictions (quantity and quality); centralized and bureaucratic administration and management; political and partisan use of health policies; the population's lack of education and awareness of health; and instability in the leadership (both institutional and community). In some countries, the situation is aggravated by different kinds of social upheaval. The three years since the previous monitoring report on health for all by the year 2000 and primary health care have witnessed armed confrontations in Nicaragua, El Salvador, and Peru; serious violent incidents in Colombia as a consequence of drug traffic; violence in Haiti in connection with the restoration of democratic order; major and far-reaching political changes in Argentina and Brazil; and transition to a democratic government in Chile.

The main obstacle—which up to now has been unpredictable because of its long duration—is the economic crisis, and it does not appear that the situation will be resolved any time soon. Not only has the crisis led to increases in unemployment and poverty, but the ensuing reduction or stagnation of per capita GNP and the weight of the external debt have influenced, through fiscal adjustment policies, the amount of resources available for both social security and health care for deprived groups. In other words, there are fewer resources to meet greater potential demand.

In light of the above, the countries have approached the development of national health policies and strategies by working toward greater efficiency in the use of their resources through decentralization and restructuring of health systems, including carrying out administrative reforms, establishing logistical and managerial systems, mobilizing resources, especially at the local level, and coordinating with sectoral or extrasectoral institutions or orientating the activities of nongovernmental organizations. As a result, community involvement has been emphasized, which can be a valuable tool for the better utilization of resources at the local level.

The crucial effort of integrating national health policies and strategies with general development policies appears to be at a critical point. Several of the reporting countries said nothing in this respect, which may indicate a possible lack of integration; the other countries report that national health policies and strategies are included in development plans and that various mechanisms (plans, cabinet, committees, etc.) have been established to coordinate global policies.

The integration of health care services and other social areas has been given special impetus in recent years, in addition to the momentum that had already been generated through the development of local health systems. This new thrust has been manifested in the creation of social emergency and social investment funds aimed at focusing social activities on the most deprived groups, who are assumed to be the most adversely affected by the crisis and economic adjustment. These are specific funds, which are usually financed from external sources and for which special administrative structures have generally been created, outside the normal administrative structures of the public ministries. They are used to finance activities related to maternal and child health, food supplements, family farms, development of small companies, employment, basic sanitation, essential drugs, etc. As yet, there has been no evaluation of their impact. Several countries have developed different projects utilizing such funds (Bolivia, Honduras, Ecuador, Jamaica, Venezuela, etc.) and several more plan to do so.

With some exceptions (Canada, the United States, Cuba, and, to a lesser degree, Costa Rica, the Bahamas, Mexico, and Venezuela), the countries report a lack of medium- and long-term plans, because they have not been able to establish long-term strategies or a political consensus for the development of health care and socioeconomic status as a whole. Without true integration and coordination, it will be difficult to maintain the rate of improvement in health that has been achieved over the last 30 years. Increasing urban poverty, lack of accessibility in rural areas, decreased domestic availability of food products, lack of progress in basic sanitation services, deterioration of public hospitals, social security problems due to losses or cuts in funding, and increasing urban violence, are some phenomena that exist in almost all the countries and that stand in the way of achievement of the goal of health for all by the year 2000.

Chapter 4

Development of health systems

Organization of the health system based on primary health care

All the countries continue to affirm their commitment to and adoption of the primary health care strategy as the main thrust for the development of their health systems. In reality, those that affirm this commitment are the Ministers or Secretaries of Public Health, but in most cases they do not represent the entire system of services, given that in recent decades social security has become increasingly important as a provider of services, primarily medical care. There are no laws that empower the Ministries to coordinate all the services and resources provided to the population. Consequently, the information reported by the countries basically covers only the services that are organized under the Ministry of Public Health. In many countries this means that only part of the population, not the majority, benefits from the measures that have been implemented to provide services based on the primary health care strategy.

Improving the coordination among the sector's institutions is a goal shared by almost all the countries. However, save for few exceptions the process is reported to be still incipient, particularly with regard to coordination of the services provided by social security institutions and those provided by Ministries of Health. Bolivia, Brazil, Costa Rica, Mexico, Panama, and Venezuela report significant advances since 1985, ranging from the formulation of a legal framework for the coordination/integration of services to the development of common technical and administrative standards among the institutions and the implementation of integrated models of multi-institutional services in pilot regions. The countries mention the following factors as obstacles to intersectoral coordination: resistance and inertia on the part of institutional bureaucracies, normative and managerial discrepancies among the institutions, differences in administrative and financial management, lack of legal standards for administrative and financial management, lack of adequate legal standards, and the large number of institutions involved. The case of Peru, where a 1985 law that provided for the integration of services was repealed, is indicative of the magnitude of the obstacles. Cuba and Canada are the two countries that have been most successful in organizing their health services on the basis of primary health care using different schemes to provide coverage for the entire population: Canada has a law providing for federal and provincial health insurance and Cuba has a single system that is administered and financed by the State.

The acceptance and inclusion of the primary health care strategy within the various levels and institutions that comprise the health sector have been achieved only partially in most of the reporting countries. Among the most frequently cited obstacles to full incorporation of the strategy are:

—the predominantly curative orientation of the health services and of many professional groups;

—insufficient physical and financial resources for health promotion and protection activities and not enough basic health teams at the primary care level;

—resistance from professional groups and institutions within the sector to fully adopt the primary health care strategy and lack of interest, knowledge, motivation, and commitment on the part of health care personnel regarding the development of such strategies;

—the trend toward a narrow interpretation of primary health care as a single program or a set of vertical programs whose components are developed separately and unequally;

—the numerous institutions involved in the health sector in many countries, which makes it difficult to achieve intersectoral coordination and establish a uniform conceptual and operational definition of the primary health care strategy; and

—the insufficient development of community involvement as a component of primary health care strategy in the majority of countries.

The countries report that various measures have been adopted to strengthen health systems, utilizing the primary health care strategy as a basis. In most countries, this process has been oriented toward strengthening services at the local level and introducing local programming schemes and intra- and intersectoral coordination mechanisms at the local and regional levels. There is a trend in many countries toward administrative schemes based on decentralization and deconcentration of management mechanisms and the regionalization of health services. In several countries, models of attention have been formulated that emphasize coordination and the most rational use of existing institutional resources at the local and regional levels. Efforts have been made to educate and train human resources to work at the primary care level and to introduce the concept of primary health care in education programs for health professionals.

In many countries, social and geographical operational criteria have been established to identify the least-served and highest-risk population groups with a view to channeling available resources to them selectively, thus achieving greater equity in the delivery of services. However, the number and exact location of these deprived groups have generally not been determined, nor have any records been kept that would make it possible to effectively evaluate the delivery of services.

In addition to the above-mentioned obstacles, there are new challenges to be overcome in the organization of health care systems based on primary health care. These include the increasingly important role of NGOs (in some areas of Haiti and Bolivia these are the only entities providing services to the population) and the creation of the Social Emergency or Social Investment Funds. The NGOs are nonpublic multisectoral institutions, and the Funds are multisectoral, although they can be held under the aegis of a public institution, usually the Ministry of Planning, or attached to the presidency. They are new actors that necessitate flexibility and adaptation on the part of health authorities in order to provide responses with a clear social impact.

The countries report that their systems of referral and back-referral of patients are not functioning smoothly and effectively in the majority of cases. This is due in part to the fact that response capacity has not been adapted at the different levels of referral. Some countries, such as Chile, Mexico, and Venezuela, have succeeded in establishing mechanisms for referral of patients with specific problems (high-risk mothers and children, AIDS, auxiliary services, diagnoses, emergencies). Guyana reports a straightforward reference system that operates with well-defined functions at five levels. In most of the countries, the incipient schemes of decentralization and development of local health systems have included patient referral as a basic point to be promoted in the near future.

Intersectoral collaboration

The reporting countries agree that practically all the national sectors involved in the process of overall development directly or indirectly affect the health status of the population. Among the most directly related sectors are agriculture; education; social welfare; protection and improvement of the environment, including water supply and basic sanitation and control of environmental pollution; housing and human settlements; employment; and population and family planning programs. In some countries, the armed forces and public safety sectors have participated by providing logistical support for national campaigns and mobilizations related to health. They also have begun to collaborate with the judicial system on problems associated with drug addiction, smoking, accidents, etc.

The sector whose basic function is to regulate the quantity of resources available for public health and other basic services involves the institutions that oversee public spending and national finances—the Treasury Ministries and the central banks. During this reporting period, most Latin American and Caribbean countries, faced with the economic crisis, established economic adjustment or reactivation policies characterized by a marked reduction in public spending on activities that are considered nonproductive, such as health and education. These policies have led to a reduction (Colombia reports a 50% reduction in the public health share of the national budget over the last 10 years), or at best a stagnation in the amount of resources available for the development and operation of health services. They have also adversely affected most of the population, limiting their access to the elements necessary to meet their most basic needs (food, employment, housing, etc.). There have been instances in which programs with a clear social and multisectoral emphasis were discontinued, as was the case with the National Food Program (PAN) in Argentina and the food program for pensioners and retirees in Uruguay.

The impact on health of these cost-containment policies and reduction in the quality of life for large sectors of the Region have not yet been examined comprehensively, but available information reveals that they have already had an effect on the health of the most vulnerable groups and will continue to do so for some time to come. It should be pointed out that the impact of reductions in multisectoral social expenditure will not necessarily be reflected in the traditional health indicators, such as mortality (infant and maternal mortality, life expectancy, etc.). The deterioration or stagnation in living conditions (especially with regard to the quality, quantity, and timely availability of food, adequate sanitation, and access to health services, etc.) of large population groups is not necessarily accompanied by a greater number of deaths.

The countries have established different institutional mechanisms in order to render the goals and activities of the various development sectors as coherent and mutually supportive among themselves and vis-à-vis the general development policy. In some, the ministers in the social area have formed a social development cabinet or council in order to formulate, enact, and evaluate coordinated policies and programs. These bodies include the Social Front in Ecuador, the Social Committee in El Salvador, the Social Investment Funds in Guatemala and Bolivia, and the National Solidarity Program (PRONASOL) in Mexico. In other countries it is the Secretariat or Ministry of Planning that is responsible for coordinating intersectoral action (Ministry of Planning and International Cooperation in Chile). The coordination mechanisms that are most often utilized are those that have been established in response to concrete problems, such as occupational health programs (work-related accidents) or educational programs (both within schools of medicine for the training of human resources and at schools in immunization or health education programs for parents and children).

Some countries have implemented intersectoral coordination mechanisms at the local and regional levels. In Guatemala, urban and rural development councils have been established, with multi-institutional and community involvement. Similar agencies at the municipal, cantonal, or district level have been instituted in Bolivia, Costa Rica, and Mexico. Other countries have had success with *ad hoc* mechanisms of interinstitutional coordination based on concrete activities or projects, such as vaccination campaigns, child survival, and water and sanitation.

In recent years, as a result of the policy of decentralization, there have been various coordination agreements between public health authorities at the central level and political authorities in smaller administrative subdivisions (state, province, department). Chile has decentralized the primary level to the *municipios*, Brazil has transferred assistance units to the municipal states, Colombia has restructured its national health system, and Uruguay has established agreements between public health authorities and the municipal governments for the primary health care services.

There are very few countries (United States, Canada, and, to a lesser extent, Cuba) that have procedures for the systematic analysis and evaluation of the repercussions of major development projects on health. However, many countries are concerned about the matter, and the environmental impact assessments required by all international and some bilateral financing agencies include evaluations of the impact of such projects on health. Already existing environmental pollution has elicited growing concern and a subsequent search for solutions, particularly in such places as Mexico City and Santiago, Chile, where the problem is so great that it has noticeably affected the population's health. But it is the impact of development in the Amazon region in Brazil that has perhaps inspired the greatest concern at both the national and international levels, not only for health reasons but because of the ecological disruption it could bring.

Noteworthy for their degree of progress are the multisectoral projects on smoking, drugs, the environment, and cities that are being carried out in Canada, in keeping with that country's priority on promotion and prevention. Environmental priorities will have their greatest expression in Canada's Green Plan.

The obstacles that stand in the way of achieving the highest possible level of intersectoral collaboration in health development are:

—insufficient consensus regarding priorities and even regarding the political and ideological framework of the various institutions and sectors in the countries, partly owing to the fact that national development plans tend not to be very specific about sectoral goals and activities;

—a scarcity of financial resources for joint intersectoral actions;

—weakness or lack of technical and administrative mechanisms for the local, multisectoral, and participatory programming of activities at the local level;

—persistence of managerial and administrative models characterized by centralization and concentration of the decision-making process, which limits local autonomy to undertake multisectoral actions;

—the low priority assigned to the health sector and its limited powers of mobilization and negotiation vis-à-vis other sectors in the country;

—a scarcity of trained human resources with intersectoral work experience, especially at the middle management level; and

—lack of political will at the highest decision-making levels to establish effective mechanisms of intersectoral coordination.

In several countries, as part of efforts to develop local health systems under a decentralized scheme, efforts are being undertaken to foster and facilitate the creation of operational mechanisms for joint programming and coordination between sectors at the local level. This is the case in Costa Rica, where the Ministry of Public Health and the Costa Rican Social Security Fund participate in the joint annual operational preparation at the local health systems level and the mechanism that is planned in Mexico, based on the modification (under study) of the General Health Law.

16

Community participation

The diversity of sociopolitical models in the Region's developing countries is reflected in the varying degree and form of community participation in health actions and in the development process. The period since the first evaluation of health for all by the year 2000 in 1985 has been characterized by the consolidation and extension of the process of democratization in the Region. Since 1988, new constitutional regimes have been established in Chile, Haiti, and Paraguay. Changes of government have come about through constitutional means in the other countries of Latin America and the Caribbean. The level and nature of community participation in health must be analyzed in the context of these overall political processes, especially in countries that have recently emerged from situations in which democratic participation in national political life was clearly restricted or limited.

All the reporting countries indicate that their stated policies acknowledge the need to support and promote community participation as an essential component in the primary health care strategy. In practice, the implementation of these policies is usually limited to community participation in isolated aspects of the execution of certain activities at the local level, especially through health collaborators or volunteers or through the contribution of labor and funds for the construction of small local infrastructure projects, particularly in the area of basic sanitation. In some countries, such as Bolivia, mechanisms have been established to allow the participation of organizations representing the communities of the country in the formulation, execution, and evaluation of policies and programs at the national level, the strategy of social management being one of the priorities of the current government. In others, such as Canada, Costa Rica, Honduras, Nicaragua, and Peru, the Ministries of Health have created programs, offices, or departments that are responsible for promoting, coordinating, and regulating community involvement in health programs. In Colombia, the Committees of Community Participation were established by presidential decree, and in Venezuela community hospital boards have been established to permit community participation in hospital establishments.

In the Bahamas, Belize, and Suriname, community involvement has mainly been handled through the NGOs. In Cuba, it is carried out through social and grass-roots organizations. In Canada it is estimated that the contribution of volunteer agencies to health and social services activities in 1990 amounted to more than one billion Canadian dollars. In Montevideo, Uruguay, area committees have been created to provide for extensive participation by the residents of the various areas. In the United States of America, in addition to work in the counties and the participation of various organizations, community involvement has occurred in the context of the Healthy People 2000 plan and the corresponding Consortium involving more than 300 organizations, which was created to assist in developing and implementing the plan. In Nicaragua, community participation was strengthened by focusing on the Campaign for the Defense of Children's Lives (Campaña por la Defensa de la Vida del Niño).

All the countries report the existence of some type of community volunteers, especially in rural areas and lately also in certain deprived urban areas. They may perform such functions as collaborating in specific programs, such as those for vector control or control of diarrheal diseases, or they may be traditional or formally trained midwives. In other countries there are community agents, trained and regularly supervised by the health service, who carry out more extensive health promotion and basic health care activities (Bolivia, Costa Rica, Ecuador, El Salvador, Guatemala, Honduras, Mexico, Peru). In some countries, mass campaigns have been organized, especially in relation to immunization activities, with community groups (boards of trustees, community groups, churches, etc.) participating in programming and execution at the local level. In the case of

Bolivia, this participation has been extended to the national level through the creation of the Popular Health Council.

In all the countries, the contribution of nongovernmental organizations (NGOs) to the development of primary health care is recognized and promoted. In some countries, the role of NGOs basically involves supporting health education and health promotion activities, while in others, NGOs act as suppliers of primary level services for a large sector of the population, especially isolated groups who are not covered by any type of official service.

In Bolivia, Guatemala, Haiti, and Honduras agreements have been made between the government and the main NGOs that provide health care services to improve coordination in the programming and execution of activities.

Among the principal obstacles to community involvement in the strategy of primary health care that have been identified by the reporting countries are:

—lack of appropriate attitude, behavior, and knowledge on the part of health care personnel with regard to promoting, supervising, and accepting community involvement in programs, and lack of human resources trained for community promotion;

—frequent shifts among community representatives and volunteers, which makes it difficult to achieve stable development and ongoing training of community resources;

—frustration generated by the limited capacity of the health services to provide an appropriate and timely response to the demands of the community;

—the population's limited knowledge of health and low educational level, as well as apathy—stemming from the inability to satisfy their basic needs—which limits their interest and capacity to participate in the programming and evaluation of actions;

—difficulties in establishing communication between the communities and the health services because of geographical inaccessibility, lack of communications media, cultural and linguistic differences, etc.;

—the situation of internal armed conflict that prevails in some countries of the Region;

—the existence of a paternalistic perspective, both in the field and among high-level authorities, that does not distinguish between community involvement and community manipulation, along with a trend toward the partisan politization of the mechanisms of community involvement;

—scarcity of the material resources necessary to effectively promote community involvement (vehicles, educational materials, etc.); and

—bureaucratic rigidity and the persistence of centralized forms of management and administration of the health services, making them less flexible and less able to provide a timely response to the demands of the participatory process.

The countries have conceived several specific short- or medium-term measures to overcome these shortfalls. In several, use of the mass media will be strengthened in order to disseminate a basic knowledge of health and promote an awareness of each person's responsibility to protect his own health and that of his family members. In addition, there will be efforts in almost all the countries to strengthen programs for health education and training of leaders at the community level. Several countries will take steps to increase awareness and improve the aptitude of health personnel regarding the promotion of community involvement. In countries that have plans to promote the development of local health systems and administrative decentralization, mechanisms will be implemented with a view to achieving community involvement in the process of local programming and other aspects of service management.

Authorities in Peru indicate that unless the above-mentioned obstacles are overcome relatively quickly in many of the countries of Latin America and unless some success is achieved in actions involving community participation, progress made thus far could be reversed, which would lead the population's interest to decrease.

Managerial process and mechanisms

In the last five years, the health services management process in most of the countries has shared some features, given the sweeping fiscal austerity and rationalization of expenditure measures that most of the countries have had to introduce. There also have been administrative reforms aimed at increasing efficiency in the public sector. Some countries have gone so far as to experiment with schemes for the partial or total transfer of certain services traditionally handled by the State to the private sector, as has been the case in Chile with the partial privatization of social security. Even in those countries that have managed to avoid the privatization of health services, considerable pressure is being exerted on the health sector to exercise greater control and obtain better results from the limited resources available. Consequently, carrying out a revision and reformulation of the administrative and managerial processes in the health services became a fundamental priority during this period.

The democratization of national political life, shared by many Latin American countries, also is marked by a trend toward deconcentration and decentralization of the State's administrative functions. In several countries, attempts are being made to strengthen regional, State, departmental, and municipal systems, in order to increase the capability of the State apparatus to respond to the demands of the population.

The health sector is not immune to this process. Most countries have attempted to create, strengthen, and reinforce local health systems as the main instrument for achieving the goal of health for all by the year 2000. In terms of the development of local health systems, the countries propose to establish the following mechanisms to increase the efficiency and operating capacity of their services:

—an effective coordination and even integration of the services provided by different institutions in and outside the sector at the local and regional levels;

—the implementation of integrated and participatory processes in the local programming of health activities with a view to facilitating an equitable, efficient, and effective utilization of the resources available to respond to the community's most urgent health priorities and problems in the community;

—the development of technical and administrative capabilities of mid-level management at the regional and local levels as a necessary prerequisite for the gradual decentralization of service management; and

—the design and establishment of information, surveillance, and evaluation systems aimed at supporting effective leadership and management in the health systems.

Several countries have reviewed and modified the sector's institutional and organic/functional framework in order to clear the way for new management schemes. Attempts have been made to strengthen the normative, regulatory, and supervisory roles of the central levels of Ministries or Secretariats of Health, in conjunction with increasing the executive functions and responsibilities of the peripheral agencies of these institutions or other agencies and organizations that are involved in the delivery of services, such as social security, municipalities, provincial governments, NGOs, etc. (Brazil, Mexico, Bahamas, Belize, and Suriname). In other countries, the responsibilities and sphere of action of the various institutions comprising the sector have been more precisely delimited as a prelude to greater intrasectoral coordination and possibly integration (Costa Rica, Panama, Venezuela).

In some countries, legal instruments and standards have been formulated and implemented as a step toward decentralized management, not only in the health sector but in other public services (Colombia, Guatemala, Mexico, Peru). Moreover, many Ministries of Health in the Region have modified their technical, policy-making, and administrative structures, in keeping with the decentralization objective and in order to facilitate the administrative and managerial processes in the priority programs; this effort, however, sometimes has been pursued following decisions made at the central level of the government—state reform in Argentina and administrative and financial state reforms in Bolivia. In order to facilitate management, several bodies have been created, including the National Advisory Council, the National Private Health Council in Chile, the National Health Council in Paraguay, the National Regionalized and Integrated Health System in Peru, the Canadian Health Committee in Canada, and the Healthy People Consortium in the United States. In Venezuela, attention on management has been channeled through a major effort aimed at maintenance and managerial training. Cuba has implemented new managerial processes based on research and technology in the areas of biotechnology, drugs, equipment, and tourism and health.

There are many obstacles to the adoption of such managerial measures, including:

—insufficient economic resources for promoting administrative decentralization, such as those needed for wage standardization;

—a scarcity of sufficiently trained managers at the peripheral level;

—a multiplicity and lack of coordination and effective control of projects that are financed by external sources, which leads to a splintering of the efforts of technical and administrative managers at the central and peripheral levels;

—a lack of coherence among policies, strategies, and operational plans of the sector's various institutions, as well as the introduction of political and partisan criteria in the distribution of resources to the institutions and peripheral levels;

—the absence of a sufficient and reliable information base for monitoring, evaluating, and supporting the administrative and managerial processes in the sector; and

—a lack of cost systems that would facilitate a more equitable and effective distribution of available resources.

For the public sector, especially public hospitals, the situation is aggravated by the lack of a real maintenance and repair program (including equipment and specialized human resources). There were many instances in which these institutions were unable to provide service to the public because they lacked basic inputs and/or their equipment had deteriorated. Moreover, as a result of the economic adjustment policies, several new hospitals (or facilities under construction) will be unable to operate because of a lack of resources. The management of the physical infrastructure currently represents a serious stumbling block. If to this one adds the fact that the traditional structure of resources (human and physical) in the public sector is out of sync with the new epidemiological profile of the population and its demands (in Argentina, Chile, Uruguay as a whole, and in many urban areas in other countries), it is clear that there are too many difficulties to be overcome for the managerial measures to produce, in the short term, any qualitative and quantitative improvement in services to the population.

Furthermore, the traditional resistance in the public sector to reassign human resources (aggravated by the increase in unemployment) will undermine any managerial measure aimed at changing the profile of health personnel.

Human resources for health

This is the area where the obstacles to progress toward the goal of health for all by the year 2000 and the implementation of the primary health care strategy can best be appreciated. While in 1988 twelve countries reported having (or being in the process of preparing) a plan for human resources in health in order to meet the needs of the primary health care strategy, there are now only two that currently have a plan (Cuba and Mexico, which already had plans in 1988) and one, the Bahamas, where one is being developed. Some countries are carrying out evaluations, particularly in order to establish some permanent registration system for health personnel (Bolivia, Honduras) or to assess the quality of the service provided by professional personnel (for example, the National Practitioner Data Bank in the United States). But the general tenor of the responses is that there is no national policy regarding the training of human resources to meet the needs of health for all and primary health care, although there are training programs for existing resources, especially nonprofessionals working at the local level.

The importance of the health sector as an employer (of the economically active population) is growing: 8% in Canada and Cuba, 7% in the United States, 4% in Argentina, and 3% in Brazil. Individual countries vary greatly, but in all of them the sector accounts for an ever-increasing proportion of the total work force. Physicians basically constitute the bulk of health personnel in the countries of Latin America. With the exception of Cuba, there are many more doctors than nurses in all the Latin American countries. The situation is reversed in the United States, Canada, and the non-Latin Caribbean, where there are more than three nurses for every doctor. And yet, in Latin America, except for Cuba, the number of nursing auxiliaries and aides is increasing. All of the above means that there is an exceptional situation regarding the supply and demand of employment in the sector, with all the consequences that this potentially has for the motivation and participation of personnel in the primary health care strategy.

Human resources training has followed the trend described above. Between 1960 and 1988, the number of schools of medicine increased from 97 to 217 in Latin America and from 98 to 144 in North America.

The employment situation of physicians varies tremendously from country to country, which necessarily brings about differences in the implementation of health for all and primary health care. On the one hand, there are countries such as Bolivia, Guatemala, Honduras, and Peru where the principal employer is the public sector (Ministry of Health), and on the other hand, there are countries such as Brazil, Costa Rica, and Mexico where the principal employer is (directly or indirectly) social security, an agency of the state. Then there is a third type of country where the principal sources of income for physicians are corporate-controlled (Argentina) or private (Uruguay) insurance firms.

Haiti continues to be the country with the lowest availability of health personnel to serve the population—some 900 physicians for a population of nearly 6 million; Bolivia, Honduras, and Guatemala follow. At the other extreme are Argentina, Cuba, and Uruguay with about 3 doctors per 1000 population, more than the United States and Canada.

Several trends appear to be developing, such as possible controls on enrollment in Argentina, Uruguay, and Mexico. In Cuba, in addition to a strict training plan for family physicians that is based on comprehensive general medicine, the decision has been made to train nursing personnel only at the university level. Canada has begun to limit enrollment and residencies in medicine because of the excessive number of doctors already available. In Chile, which reports no personnel problems in relation to primary health care requirements, there is a need to cover 12,000 currently vacant positions in the National Health System. In the United States, control is exercised through monitoring of professional performance. In Haiti, as a result of economic crisis and institutional instability, the training of auxiliary personnel has been suspended.

There has been no analysis nor is there any methodology for studying progress toward a more equitable distribution of human resources. Available information indicates that there is a greater concentration of personnel in urban centers than in rural areas. Haiti reports that the distribution worsened after 1988; the main reasons reported for this situation are the economic crisis, limited financial resources, and the reluctance of health personnel to move to the least developed areas.

Several countries have instituted or strengthened training programs for training professional and mid-level health personnel, using a teaching-service approach as a way to expose medical and nursing students and mid-level technicians, at the outset of their training, to the concepts and practice of primary health care in the primary level services in an extramural, community context. Many countries report having recently carried out curriculum revisions in their professional training programs in order to incorporate more elements of public health and the primary health care strategy, as well as establishing programs or schools to train specialists in public health and health services administration. Some have particularly emphasized the training of teaching personnel. All the countries have some program to provide continuing education for health personnel in specific aspects of the primary health care strategy. Several have created interinstitutional commissions of human resources for health care in order to improve coordination and planning in this area.

Most of the countries report that the main obstacles to improving the availability of human resources for primary health care stem from the current economic-financial crisis. Salaries in the majority of the countries are insufficient to overcome the reluctance of professionals to move to rural or relatively inaccessible areas. The lack of supplies, infrastructure, and basic equipment in underserved areas is a source of frustration, and leads health care workers to flee these services. The absence of any clear national policies or plans for training health personnel, along with the consequent lack of coordination and efficiency in the use of the resources available for this purpose, has helped worsen the situation in several countries.

Research and technology

Very few of the reporting countries indicate having any national policy on health research and technology (even if merely stated or only in the early stages of application).

The development and maintenance of scientific and technical infrastructure is an area in which the gap between the Latin American and Caribbean countries and the developed world has, in general, widened. Most of the countries in the Region have not even come close to the goal of devoting 1% of their GDP for research and development, as advocated by the United Nations; in fact, they seem to have moved in the opposite direction in recent years, with the exception of Cuba, which is implementing an ambitious program that emphasizes biotechnology, drugs, and equipment. The most notable example of the decline in research and technology is Argentina, where there has been a new wave of emigration among investigators. This "brain drain" toward developed countries, especially to the United States, has been particularly pronounced in the Region.

Given the size of their populations and their level of economic-productive development, most countries have not been able to achieve the critical mass that would enable them to initiate and sustain research and development programs. Moreover, the government authorities' lack of political vision during the last few decades, and their failure to invest in this type of activity, has not helped the situation.

At this point, more emphasis is being placed on the study and rationalization of the technology currently available than on research and/or the creation of local technology. In keeping with this focus, several countries have established a basic institutional capacity for action in this area through the creation of vice ministries, departments, institutions, centers, nuclei, and programs for health technology (Argentina, Brazil, Colombia, Costa Rica, Cuba, Chile, Ecuador, Mexico, Uruguay, Venezuela). These entities generally produce reviews and inventories of the existing technology in the country, which are then used to prepare priority lists of needed technologies that can serve as markers so that the regulatory institutions in every sector can establish specific guidelines. The coordination of health technology's selection and use generally is poorly developed in most of the countries. In some, this function is assigned to commissions, academies, national ministries of science and technology, or specific interinstitutional groups, but almost all the reporting countries indicate deficiencies in this area, and certain initiatives, such as INDES in Peru, have been discontinued. In the United States, however, many of the health for all by the year 2000 goals and objectives have come out of the National Institutes of Health, the foremost health research center in that country. And in Mexico, the Instituto Nacional de Salud (INS) is making important contributions to the new health policy.

In terms of identifying and developing research proposals that focus on priority health problems, eight countries have explicit guidelines and five are in the process of formulating them. The approaches utilized correspond to priorities derived from the epidemiological profile and level of development of the health services: basic applied clinical and epidemiological research on the most prevalent infectious, contagious, and parasitic diseases; food and nutrition problems; human reproduction; alcoholism and drug addiction; traffic accidents; chronic and prevalent diseases; and AIDS. Several countries have instituted guidelines for establishing priorities in health services research and associated technologies, such as drug production, natural medicine, and epidemiology applied to the planning, administration, and training of human resources.

In nine countries, the coordination, promotion, and dissemination of health research results are the responsibility of national health institutes or interinstitutional national research commissions; the others lack formal mechanisms for this purpose. The countries mentioned several factors that have impeded the effective development and application of policies in health research and technology, including the perennial problem of insufficient financial resources for investment in research on priority concerns, lack of sufficient trained investigators and infrastructure, weak mechanisms of interinstitutional coordination for the rational utilization of resources for research, and lack of political will to promote research as an instrument of development.

In order to offset these difficulties, the countries plan to establish or strengthen the leading agencies in health science and technology so they can coordinate, promote, and disseminate the efforts that are being carried out in this area and make specific allocations for research in the budgets of the institutions in the sector. Several countries intend to mount efforts to sensitize the political authorities and the public to the need to view the development of science and technology as an essential component in general and sectoral development.

Resource utilization and mobilization

Of the reporting countries, only four indicated that they had a basic plan for the mobilization and use of material and financial resources in support of the national strategy of health for all by the year 2000 (Cuba, Mexico, Canada, and the United States).

Most of the countries have reassigned resources toward deprived areas and groups, especially through the above-mentioned emergency funds and through several special programs related to the local health systems and national policies of decentralization and deconcentration of services. Bolivia reports the existence of 94 districts organized as local health systems. Chile has prepared, with international support, an investment plan for 1990–1991 to address major financing and maintenance problems in the hospital network, and it is also carrying out a program to strengthen primary health care in 24 urban and 104 rural high-risk areas.

According to IDB and World Bank data, the domestic economic resources mobilized at the central government level for health care during the period 1980–1989 either remained the same or increased in the United States, Cuba, Canada, Belize, Chile, Ecuador, Honduras, and Venezuela; in the other 16 countries they decreased. Colombia reported that the central government's share diminished 50%. It would be necessary to undertake a country-by-country study in order to fully analyze this phenomenon, since, as a result of decentralization and state reforms, income that previously corresponded to the central government is now collected at the departmental level (in Bolivia, for example). This has affected the manner in which resources are distributed among the sectors by authorities of the central government. The reduction in central government spending began in the late 1980s; however, the studies that have been carried out would appear to indicate that priority programs have been maintained (EPI, Maternal and Child Health, etc.) and that the principal impact has been a decline in the quality of hospital care (lack of maintenance and repair and scarcity of inputs), along with a drop in the real wages of health care workers.

There is a lack of organization, standards, and information on the source, utilization, amount, and status of the various resources (human and physical), especially regarding the economic aspects of service delivery, and this continues to be one of the major obstacles to monitoring and evaluating health programs.

In several countries steps have been taken to increase efficiency in the utilization and productivity of available resources through the establishment of expenditure, production, and cost systems; streamlined administrative procedures; a managerial approach for information systems; and other measures. Attempts also have been made to mobilize more resources from state, municipal, or provincial entities in support of the process of decentralization and strengthening of local health systems.

The most prevalent obstacles to the mobilization of resources include the fiscal crisis, excessive external indebtedness, domestic inflation, higher prices for basic inputs in the international market, wage losses, and increased unemployment.

The countries' reporting regarding their expenditures on health has improved, with 19 countries covering this component in their reports; the data, however, are not comparable, since they are calculated on according to different bases. Argentina, Costa Rica, the United States, Uruguay, Brazil, Suriname, Peru, Chile, and Belize reported on total expenditure as a percentage of GNP, while the Bahamas, Bolivia, El Salvador, Guyana, Honduras, Jamaica, Nicaragua, and Paraguay presented public sector expenditure. Mexico included social security information, and Cuba's data were based on its own GNP accounting. The fact that it is not known whether reported government expenditure corresponded only to the central government or to the government in general posed an additional complication. The proportion of national expenditures allocated to primary health care is even more difficult to determine because some countries report only on expenditure for specific programs of coverage extension without including, for example, outpatient care, health education, and environmental improvement services. Most of the countries report that they are unable to calculate what they spend on primary health care. This situation reflects a lack or deficiency of information in the countries regarding the production, costs, and expenditures of the services by level of care, without which it is almost impossible to objectively monitor the efficiency and equity of resource distribution and allocation.

Chapter 5

International action

International movement of resources

Few countries have carried out systematic analyses of the needs for international cooperation in relation to the national health for all by the year 2000 strategy; those that had did so a number of years ago. The best efforts in this area have been those carried out with the Organization's support in the Central American countries, Panama, and the Dominican Republic. Since 1984, these countries have participated in the Plan for Priority Health Needs in Central America and Panama, and have jointly systematized their requirements for external financial cooperation in six priority areas through the development of a common portfolio of national and subregional projects. Since 1985, under this initiative, the Central American countries have succeeded in mobilizing a total of US$390,000,000 from external sources for health development in the subregion. The second stage of this plan was presented at an international meeting in May 1991.

The number of different agencies, governments, international agencies, NGOs, foundations, religious associations, etc., that carry out actions or provide funds for activities directly or indirectly related to health is very large and increasing. Other than the control and coordination mechanisms that exist for these entities, there is no information on the true magnitude of international action. The countries' reports basically cover those projects that are under the responsibility of the Ministries of Health or other ministries, and there is very little information on the economic volume of these projects.

In general, what exists is a list of priorities that includes all the components of the primary health care strategy (water and basic sanitation, immunization and infant survival, maternal health and family planning, control of communicable diseases, food and nutrition, essential drugs and development of the pharmaceutical industry, control of chronic diseases), as well as projects aimed at increasing the operating capacity of the health services by enhancing the capacity of the physical installations and infrastructure, maintenance of installations and equipment, training of human resources, development of biotechnology, and strengthening of the managerial system.

Inter-country cooperation

Almost all the reporting countries have established cooperation agreements to promote joint health actions in border areas, especially regarding vector-borne disease control, immunization activities, and epidemiological surveillance. There also are bilateral or multilateral agreements involving several countries for the purpose of exchanging knowledge and experiences and carrying out joint research and manpower training in specific areas of common interest such as biotechnology, drug production and quality control, nutrition education, and prevention of drug addiction and rehabilitation of addicts.

The most important mechanism of technical cooperation among countries in recent years has been the Plan for Priority Health Needs in Central America and Panama, which not only has mobilized external resources but has also served as a means of achieving closer technical cooperation between the countries of the subregion in areas of mutual interest and priority such as malaria control, food and nutrition, training of human resources, infant survival, and essential drugs. This process of cooperation and collaboration between the Central American countries has developed rapidly, despite the conflict and instability that have prevailed in the subregion during this period, which makes it all the more remarkable. Several annual meetings of subregional health authorities have already been held. The countries that participate in this plan are Belize, Costa Rica, El Salvador, Guatemala, Honduras, Nicaragua, Panama, and the Dominican Republic. As an off-shoot of this experience, these same countries have crafted another subregional project—the Social Investment Program for the Development of the Central American Isthmus. In South America, the Andean Cooperation in Health has been further strengthened through the Hipólito Unanue Agreement.

Canada and the United States have had agreements to cooperate on bilateral activities for many years. Cuba has recently signed bilateral accords with Belize, Bolivia, Guyana, Peru, and the Dominican Republic, and has pending agreements with Argentina, Brazil, Ecuador, and Venezuela. These agreements deal with cooperation in human resources, maintenance, technology, and rehabilitation.

As a result of the MERCOSUR agreement (Argentina, Brazil, Paraguay, and Uruguay), Brazil and Argentina have signed various cooperation agreements on drugs and medications.

International technical cooperation

The Organization's cooperation with the countries of the Region is considered useful for the development of the various components of the primary health care strategy; in all, support has been received in the form of national and international technical advisory services, manpower training within and outside the country, dissemination of scientific and technical information, the strengthening of national capacity to coordinate international cooperation in health and mobilize additional external resources, the promotion of research applied to the priority problems of the country, and the contribution of financial resources for specific activities of importance.

Several countries indicated that these subregional cooperation initiatives also have helped to improve the utilization of the Organization's technical cooperation resources. In terms of obstacles to the best possible utilization of available resources, the countries point to difficulties experienced by national programs in clearly defining their requirements for technical cooperation, as well as the frequent turnover of technical personnel in management positions, which leads to shifts in cooperation priorities and to an inadequate understanding of the Organization's role as an entity of technical, rather than financial, cooperation. On the other hand, several countries pointed out that coordination between the international agencies providing cooperation in health is frequently inadequate.

The reporting countries received technical cooperation from other agencies within the United Nations system, including UNICEF, UNDP, UNFPA, WFP, and FAO. At the bilateral level, there has been collaboration with USAID (U.S.), JICA (Japan), GTZ (Germany), Italy, France, Spain, the European Economic Community (EEC), and others. The Inter-American Development Bank (IDB) and the World Bank are assuming a leadership role not only in financial terms but also by developing important technical assistance projects in the social sectors.

In most countries, the coordination of overall international cooperation falls under the responsibility of the Secretariat or Ministry of Planning; few countries report having established offices or units within the Ministry of Health to effectively coordinate all the international cooperation in the health field.

Chapter 6

Availability of primary health care

The quantification of primary health care coverage is considered to be conceptually and methodologically complex; for the most part, the countries have responded qualitatively, reporting an improvement in the availability and accessibility of services, but without being able to express it in quantitative terms for a specific period. Few countries have provided numerical values, and in some instances, the numbers they have reported—as is the case of Mexico with 94% of the population covered by primary health care—are much higher than the figures for the individual primary health care components (basic sanitation; prenatal care, deliveries, and care of nursing infants; immunization; drugs; use of contraceptives; etc.).

The essential elements of primary health care continue to show a positive trend on the whole, although in some cases progress is very slow, such as in sanitation.

At the outset of the International Drinking Water Supply and Sanitation Decade, the Latin American and Caribbean countries were enjoying relatively good drinking water supply and sanitation services compared with other regions of the world. During the 1980s, public services in the urban sector in general were well organized, especially in terms of services for citizens in the middle- and upper-income brackets. The rural and periurban populations, however, were increasingly neglected. In addition, the situation among the poor worsened in the course of the Decade.

Given the increase in the urban population, drinking water supply and sanitation services are, in relative terms, declining. The public utility companies, many of which are economically weak, do not have the necessary incentive to extend their services to low-income and marginal areas of the cities, where the potential for recovering their costs is low. As a result, most of the poor urban population purchase their drinking water from vendors, who charge up to 35% more than the urban water supply systems.

In 1988, 55% of the rural population in Latin America had easy access, whereas 56 million people living in these areas still lacked drinking water. In the Caribbean the situation is better, but even so, 1.7 million rural inhabitants have no easy access to this vital element. In 1988, 12% of the urban population of Latin America, or around 34 million people, did not have easy access to drinking water.

The urban population that benefited from water supply services increased from 186 million (84%) in 1980 to 257.8 million (88%) in 1988, and coverage by sewerage services increased from 100 million (44%) in 1980 to 142 million (49%) in 1988. Water supply in the rural sector expanded from 49 million (40%) to 68 million (55%), and coverage by rural sanitation services reached 32% in 1988.

There are significant differences within the countries in terms of the services and the progress achieved. The urban sector enjoys better water and sanitation services, with better coverage for water than for sanitation. In 1987, four countries reported that overall coverage was under 50%, and ten reported that coverage was under 50% in the rural population. An evaluation carried out in 1985 indicated that, of the 24 countries that set water supply goals for the rural sector, 12 appeared to be close to achieving them or to have good possibilities of doing so, and 12 needed to expand their efforts significantly in order to reach their goals.

The progress achieved in expanding coverage during the first eight years of the 1980s was not as notable as had been expected, and it will not be possible to reach the target established for urban water supply (91%) in 1990; nor will it be possible to attain the target set for urban sanitation with sewerage connections (71%). The increase in water supply coverage in the rural sector, in turn, would have to be 1% greater in order to meet the target.

In most of the systems, operation and maintenance activities do not receive the necessary attention. The institutions responsible for managing water and sanitation operate basically as construction companies, and, accordingly, they emphasize construction and repairs. Resources allocated for the maintenance of infrastructure are devoted to corrective measures and only rarely to preventive maintenance. The reliance on imported equipment and parts aggravates maintenance problems at this time of scarce foreign exchange in most of the countries, leading to frequent service interruptions.

During 1990, immunization coverage using the program's vaccines reached the highest levels ever achieved in the Americas: no vaccine had coverage lower than 70%, and several of the subregions, such as the countries of the English-speaking Caribbean and those of the Southern Cone, achieved 80% or higher.

This enormous progress is mainly due to the political and social commitment that has caused high priority to be given to immunization programs in all the countries of the Americas, within PAHO itself, and in national and international collaborating agencies. Vaccination sweeps, vaccination days, and the vaccination activities carried out in the health services also have contributed to this achievement. The high level of coordination achieved between the governments and the agencies supporting immunization activities in the Western Hemisphere (USAID, UNICEF, Rotary, IDB, the Canadian Public Health Association, and PAHO) has enabled efficient and creative programs to be carried out with the best possible utilization of available resources.

The improvements obtained in all the performance indicators, such as the increased number of health units included in the weekly surveillance system—almost 20 000 at present—and the increased proportion of cases to which a final diagnosis is assigned (now 95%), are impressive. There is also an increase in the number of *municipios* with coverage above 80%—almost 60% of the 7408 *municipios* for which information is available.

Nonetheless, problems remain. Of greatest importance is the quality of monitoring the wild poliovirus being carried out based on the analysis of fecal samples from patients with acute flaccid paralysis and their contacts. The apparent progress of this activity is deceptive: in 48% of the cases reported during 1990, only two adequate and timely samples were taken and sent to the laboratory.

Highest priority is assigned to the elimination of what appear to be the last foci of infection of wild poliovirus. The Andean region is of particular concern and requires urgent attention. In addition, several foci undoubtedly exist on the Pacific and Atlantic coasts of Colombia, and the neighboring areas of Venezuela and Ecuador are at special risk. Intensive measures are recommended, especially in Colombia, where apparently vaccination campaigns have not been as comprehensive as they should have been in terms of their intensity or their scope.

There also are foci in areas of northern Peru that border on Ecuador, and it is possible that some also exist elsewhere in the country. It has been acknowledged that Peru currently suffers serious problems, including social and political disturbances and the cholera epidemic. There appears to be a need for a global program in this area, such as the one recently carried out in Central America, that would cover Peru, Ecuador, Colombia, and neighboring areas of Venezuela.

The efforts to eliminate measles in Cuba and the English-speaking Caribbean are paving the way for the implementation of effective strategies for controlling and eliminating this disease. The low coverage among priority population groups remains the leading obstacle to the control of measles, and efforts to increase coverage among children under 2 should be intensified.

As of December 1988, the estimated rate of access to oral rehydration salts in Latin America and the Caribbean was 65%, the rate of oral rehydration therapy use was 41%, and that of oral rehydration salts, 25%. This represented a considerable increase compared with the rates estimated for 1985—44%, 10%, and 10%, respectively. By 1988, 11 countries reported a rate of access to oral rehydration salts of more than 80%, and 13 countries reported a rate of 50%, reaching the regional target that had been set for 1989 (the Organization's Plan for Diarrheal Disease Control for 32 countries). Currently, 18 countries produce oral rehydration salts; local production meets national needs in 8 countries, and in 13 countries private manufacturers supply oral rehydration salts to the national programs. Thanks to production in the countries, packets of oral hydration salts are beginning to be available in pharmacies, and physicians are beginning to be encouraged to prescribe them. The regular and ongoing implementation of measures to ensure effective quality control and the availability and adequate distribution of oral hydration salts is a very important factor.

Regarding the immunization of pregnant women with tetanus toxoid, it was impossible to draw an overall comparison for this period because of the recent introduction of the indicator and the scarcity of information. Among the reporting countries, 16 supplied information in some form during the last three-year period. When these figures are compared with the values reported in the 1988 monitoring, the countries that provided information in both exercises show no significant progress: those that had low coverage remain so.

In terms of basic maternal and child health activities, most of the countries are still far behind in having permanent records that can be used for regular monitoring and evaluation of progress and/or problems. Several countries only report public sector activities, mainly those in public hospitals. Several countries do not report prenatal care, medical care at delivery, or care for nursing infants. The figures reported correspond to the years 1988, 1989, and 1990, and they represent progress by comparison with the 1988 report, which provided values from as far back as 1983. Despite reservations as to the quality and comparability of the data, as noted above, it can be said that, save for few exceptions, the picture is rather discouraging regarding progress in the coverage of pregnancy and deliveries; some of the countries say as much in their reports (Haiti and Jamaica). Brazil, Colombia, Ecuador, Jamaica, Mexico, and Suriname report less prenatal coverage than three years ago, and only Bolivia shows definite progress (from 17% to 38%). Regarding delivery coverage, Argentina, Costa Rica, Ecuador, Guatemala, Haiti, Honduras, and Mexico report lower figures, and only Bolivia and Venezuela report definite increases.

In the area of drugs and biologicals, there were advances in the 1980s, despite some problems of continuity. Of particular note are the Latin American Network of Drug Quality Control Laboratories, the ABREMEX agreement (Argentina, Brazil, Mexico, Spain), and the Revolving Drug Fund (1986, for Central America and Panama). At the country level, steps were taken to rationalize the use and prescription of drugs. A fundamental achievement was the recent creation of uniform basic tables for use by the public sector at the national level in more than 50% of the Latin American and Caribbean countries. Twelve new national drug information centers have been established and developed. On the other hand, most of the countries still lack systematic programs for drug monitoring. The programs have not been sufficient to meet the needs, nor has accessibility to low-income sectors improved, a problem due especially to rising prices.

National production of biologicals varies from country to country. Canada, the United States, and Mexico have the capability to produce all the EPI vaccines needed, and the first two are self-sufficient. On the other hand, Central America and the Caribbean, with the exception of Cuba, do not have facilities for vaccine production, and in South America some of the countries have the capability, but only meet 50% of their needs. In 1989, only two countries—Brazil and Mexico—produced vaccines for the EPI in Latin America.

It is estimated that in 1990 Latin America and the Caribbean will have approximately 15 million live newborns and 18 million pregnant women. The estimated needs and the nominal and real capacity to produce EPI vaccines for Latin America and the Caribbean (in millions of doses) are as follows:

	Needs	Nominal capacity	Real capacity
Polio	53	30	14
Measles	24	18	14
DPT	70	33	14
TT	50	26	14
BCG	30	30	26

Except in the case of BCG, Latin America and the Caribbean have a long way to go, not only to make efficient use of installed capacity, but also to achieve autonomy in meeting needs.

Chapter 7

Health status and living conditions

Population

The population of the Americas was approximately 331 million in 1950; it had already reached 729 million in 1990, and is expected to reach slightly more than 835 million by the year 2000. The Americas have approximately 13.7% of the world's population, with a mildly downward trend. Within the Hemisphere, Latin America contributes the largest percentage, accounting for 57.4% of the total in 1980. It is expected that, despite the declining birth rate noted in some of the countries, the proportion will stand at 63.2% by the year 2000. North America's share will decline from 41% to 35.3%, and that of the Caribbean from 1.6% to 1.5%.

In Latin America, Brazil stands out with a total population of just over 147 million inhabitants in 1989, followed by Mexico with almost 87 million, Argentina and Colombia with 32 million, Peru with 22 million, and Venezuela with something over 19 million. Of the 20 countries in the Region, six account for 339 million of the total population of 429 million and the remaining 90 million are distributed among the other 14 countries.

Demographic transition

Based on the combined formulation of mortality and birth rates that serves to define natural population increase, the Region's countries can be classifed into four groups, according to their stage within the demographic transition.

Group 1. Countries that combine a high birth rate with a high death rate—Bolivia and Haiti. These countries are in the early stage of demographic transition, in which mortality has begun to decline and major changes in fertility are not yet observed. The latest data from Bolivia's National Population and Health Survey, however, show that this country is making clear progress in the transition, with general fertility at 4.9 for 1984–1989 and infant mortality at 96 per 1,000 for 1979–1989.

Group 2. Countries that combine a high birth rate with a moderate death rate—El Salvador, Guatemala, Honduras, Nicaragua, Paraguay, and Peru. In this stage there is a slightly greater decline in mortality with few variations in the birth rate, which produces a relatively high growth rate.

Group 3. Countries that combine a moderate birth rate with a low death rate—Brazil, Chile, Colombia, Costa Rica, the Dominican Republic, Ecuador, Guyana, Jamaica, Mexico, Panama, Suriname, Trinidad and Tobago, Venezuela, the Windward Islands and other Caribbean territories. Most of the Region's countries are in this phase of transition, representing 45% of the population of the Americas and three-fourths that of Latin America.

Group 4. Countries that combine a low birth rate with a moderate death rate—Argentina, Barbados, Canada, Cuba, Guadeloupe, Martinique, Puerto Rico, the United States of America, and Uruguay. This group includes the countries of Latin America and the Caribbean that have come furthest in the transition process, plus the two most developed countries in the Hemisphere.

These countries have average crude death rates that are higher than those of Group 3, or even similar to those of Group 2, which are at earlier stages of transition. This effect is due to the particular age distribution of the population, which is characterized by a larger proportion of elderly due to the decline in fertility and the lengthening lifespan.

The historical evolution of birth and death rates in the demographic transition process also implies changes over time in the age distribution of the population. For each given combination of changes in the birth and death rates there is a different relative distribution of the age groups in the population.

As might be expected, the general trend as countries move to a more advanced stage of the transition, is for the percentage of children and young people to decline and the proportion of elderly to increase. One exception may be the fact that the proportion of children and young people increases slightly as a country goes from Group 1 to Group 2. This is due to reductions in infant mortality, which compensate for what is probably a moderate decline in the birth rate.

As of 1990, it has been estimated that in the countries at the beginning stages of transition, 15% of the population is under 5 years of age and just over 3% is 65 or older, whereas in the more "aged" countries, 7% of the population is in the 0–4 year group and 13% is elderly.

The effects of the current transition process on the age distribution of the population will be seen many years from now. For example, by the year 2025 Brazil may have doubled the current percentage of elderly persons in its population, but even so, this proportion group will be lower than that seen in present levels in the countries of Group 4.

The relative age distribution of the population shows little sensitivity in the short and medium term. The impact of demographic changes is seen more notably in the absolute numbers of the population and in the growth rates of the various age groups. The most significant changes occur in countries in the second and third stages of transition. Brazil, for example, will see an increase in the next decade of about half a million in the 0–4 age group, but in the same period, the population 65 and older will increase by more than 2.5 million—that is, 2.4% for the first age group compared to 39% for the second. The group of children under 5 will grow at an average annual rate of 0.2%, while the rate for those 65 and older will be 3.2%.

Fertility

In the Americas as a whole, fertility began to undergo a major decline in 1960–1965. General fertility went from values as high as or higher than 6 children per woman to 3.6 in 1985–1990; this trend suggests that the rate may fall to 3.1 by the end of the century.

Of the countries with high fertility in 1960–1965, only four still show this characteristic (Bolivia, Guatemala, Honduras, and Nicaragua). Another four (El Salvador, Haiti, Paraguay, and Peru) now have moderately high fertility, and the remaining eight countries that belonged to this group (Brazil, Colombia, Costa Rica, the Dominican Republic, Ecuador, Mexico, Panama, and Venezuela) now have levels that are moderately low. The remaining countries that currently have low fertility had a more heterogeneous pattern of fertility in the past. Those that previously had high and moderately high fertility included Chile and countries of the Caribbean; those that had low and moderately low rates included Argentina, Canada, the United States of America, and Uruguay. The above factors indicate that most of the countries of the Region show unmistakable signs of having entered the transition phase in terms of fertility.

As can be expected, in all cases the greatest contribution to total fertility comes from persons in the middle age groups, between 20 and 34 years old. This contribution ranged between 69% and 78% for the five-year period 1985–1990. However, a relatively high proportion of births still occurs among women who are considered at high risk and those under 20 or over 34 years of age. The proportion of births contributed by these women has begun to fall, but in most of the countries it is still between 25% and 30%.

The group of high-risk women is made up of two very different sectors. In the past, the contribution of women aged 35 years and older was, in most cases, higher than that of younger women. The opposite was true, however, in 1985–1990; the contribution of the latter relative to total fertility has clearly declined along with the decline in fertility, irrespective of the current level of fertility in the countries.

Fertility in women under 20 years of age, or adolescent fertility, is of special interest because of its social consequences and because of the negative impact on the health of young mothers and their children. It occurs within a context of changing sexual attitudes and behaviors, greater exposure to sexually transmitted diseases, and a rise in the age at first marriage, all of which, in turn, can lead to the increasingly frequent use of abortion to terminate unwanted pregnancies.

In all the countries, a reduction in fertility has paralleled increased urbanization. However, accumulated empirical evidence invariably points to an inverse relationship between fertility and education that is at least as significant as the relationship observed between fertility and place of residence.

Among more educated women, fertility may be as low as one-third or one-fourth the rate in uneducated women. It appears, however, that the decline in fertility has taken place mainly in the less educated groups and that this decline decreases as years of schooling increase.

It is believed that abortion continues to be the main fertility control mechanism used throughout the world, although a lack of information makes it difficult to quantify the phenomenon. In the Americas, abortion is legal only in Canada, Cuba, and the United States of America. In these countries there are no legal obstacles to the procedure, although there may be social, economic, and administrative obstacles, or even questions of interpretation related to laws and administrative practices, such as the recent United States Supreme Court decision that barred physicians working in institutions that receive federal funds from performing any type of abortion procedure or even discussing the subject at the patient's request. In countries such as Argentina and Peru, abortion is permitted only in specific medical and social circumstances; in others, such as Costa Rica, it is only permitted in order to safeguard the health of the mother, and it is only allowed in life-threatening situations in Brazil, Chile, Colombia, and Mexico. But in the vast majority of the countries the illegal status of abortion, which turns a safe surgical procedure into a dangerous one, is more theoretical than practical. In Latin America, for example, abortion has always been widely practiced, although unfortunately in a rather unsanitary manner. According to an estimate by the International Planned Parenthood Federation, Latin America and the Caribbean had one of the highest abortion rates in the world in the 1970s: one in every four pregnancies was terminated by induced abortion. To the extent that restrictive legislation remains on the books and an obscurantist attitude prevails toward abortion and contraception, without any genuine public discussion or dissemination of information, it is not surprising that, because of this and other factors, several countries have seen an increase in fertility and abortion among women aged 15–19.

Thanks to the pressure of forces such as urbanization, expanded educational opportunities, changes in women's status, and the work of family planning programs, information on contraceptives has been disseminated in the countries of the Americas. According to studies carried out in various countries, more than 75%, and in many cases more than 90%, of ever-married women of reproductive age were familiar with some contraceptive method. Over the past 10 years it appears that most countries for which there is information available have seen an increase in the use of contraceptives.

Mortality

In Latin America, life expectancy at birth increased from approximately 50 years after World War II to 67 years in 1990. In this subregion, the risk of death among children is several times lower than it was 50 years ago, and in some countries (and in areas within other countries) it is only one-tenth as high as before. Adult mortality also has decreased.

The overall and significant reduction in mortality in the Americas over the last 40 years has started at different points in the different subregions. The group of Latin American countries has gained 15 years in life expectancy at birth, starting from 51.8 years in 1950–1955. An average increase of approximately two years per five-year period has brought this figure to its current level of 66.6 years. The non-Latin Caribbean has made similar advances, with the difference that in 1950–1955 it already held an advantage of approximately 5 years of life; this advantage continues in the present, with life expectancy currently standing at 72.4 years. In North America, average life expectancy at birth was already 69.1 years four decades ago. The subsequent advances have been smaller, as might be expected at this lower level of mortality, but life expectancy at birth nonetheless reached 76.1 years in 1985–1990.

The different trends described above have produced a substantial reduction in the mortality gap among the American subregions, which have differing levels of development. For Latin America the difference with respect to North America declined from 17.3 to 9.5 years between 1950–1955 and 1985–1990, and for the non-Latin Caribbean, from 12.7 to only 3.7 years.

These advances should not cause us to lose sight of the need to further advance in reducing mortality in Latin America, where the current level corresponds to that which existed in the United States of America approximately 40 years ago (1945–1950). On the other hand, despite all the technological progress in the health field, the reduction in mortality over the last 35 years in Latin America is similar in magnitude to that which took place in the United States between 1910–1915 and 1945–1950—in other words, one that took place in an equivalent time period and that started with the same life expectancy at birth, but before the availability of most modern advances in the prevention and treatment of many diseases. In terms of the many other factors that affect health—health infrastructure; the quantity, quality, density, and distribution of health personnel; the general infrastructure (transportation, water, sanitation, communications, etc.); the degree and stability of a given political organization and in particular the relative authority of the State (for example, as regards legislation on public hygiene); the amount and distribution of income; educational levels; the physical accessibility of services; housing; diet; etc.—Latin America in 1990 still has levels that are lower, on average, than those that prevailed in the United States 40 years ago. In other words, progress in reducing mortality has been relatively greater than progress in improving other aspects of living conditions. Reduced mortality, and, thus, increased life expectancy at birth, has occurred in all the countries of the Region, despite the heterogeneity of their initial levels.

These values are based on each nation's total population. Of course, the different countries show marked differences in survival among the various social groups, but this does not necessarily mean that the gains have been concentrated exclusively in the privileged socioeconomic groups of the society, leaving behind the majority of the population. On the contrary: wherever there has been a substantial gain in life expectancy at birth at the national level, the greatest advances have occurred precisely in those social groups that have lower standards of living, which make up most of the population.

The evolution of life expectancy at birth discussed above is closely associated with the changes taking place in mortality among infants under 1 year of age. Since high mortality goes hand in hand

34

with high fertility, the exposed populations are numerically important, and mortality in the first year of life becomes a significant component in the total number of deaths. In higher-mortality countries the deaths among children under 1 year may exceed 30% of all mortality. The relative importance that mortality can have in our societies becomes apparent from an analysis of the life tables, which shows, for different ages, the relationship between years actually lived and the additional years that a person might have lived if there had been no mortality (percentage of potential life lived). For example, the years left to live in Bolivia for those in the first year of life is similar to the figure in Canada for those aged 75.

An analysis of past trends indicates that considerable advances have been made in the second half of this century, even though the subregions are at different phases in their transition to greater survival after infancy. Latin America has reduced its infant mortality rate from 127 per 1000 to the current level of 55 per 1000, with average drops of 10 points per five-year period until recently, when the decline has begun to taper off. The non-Latin Caribbean already held the advantage in 1950–1955, with a rate of 83 per 1000, which by 1970–1975 had fallen to one-half and now stands at 21 per 1000. So far, very few Latin American countries have reached this level. North America is at a very different stage in this process, and the figures for that subregion primarily reflect trends in infant mortality in the United States of America. The level in 1950–1955 was 29 per 1000 and declined in small increments (1 or 2 points every five years) during the 1950s, a trend that accelerated in the 1960s and 1970s. The five-year rate in 1985–1990 is estimated at 10 per 1000, exceeding that of some countries in other regions of the world.

The gap in infant mortality that existed between Latin America and North America has substantially narrowed in the last 40 years, from almost 100 to only 45 points. This is a notable achievement considering the periods of economic and social crisis that have occurred during this time. However, the gap that must still be overcome is sizable. If current trends are maintained in the future, the infant mortality rate that Latin America is expected to achieve in the five-year period 2020–2025—that is, almost 35 years from now—is the rate that the United States of America had 30 years ago, in 1955–1960, representing a time lag of more than half a century. Thus, it appears that the less developed countries in the Americas face the pressing task of speeding up their advances in infant survival—a task that is linked not only to the effectiveness of specific interventions but even more to the improvement in various aspects of economic and social development, where the time lag also is very large. Past experience suggests that even in those countries where the decline in infant mortality has been acceptable, the deterioration or stagnation of socio-economic development can interrupt these advances in the medium or long term.

In order to facilitate the analysis of how change occurs in the age distribution of mortality in the countries, a model has been prepared based on the historical experience of two Latin American countries—Costa Rica and Cuba—in which life expectancy at birth has reached a high level. The model was constructed by estimating the rates for different ages in each of these countries when they achieved life expectancies at birth of 50, 55, 60, 65, 70, and 75 years. These rates were averaged, and it was verified that this accurately represents the age distribution of mortality observed in the countries of Latin America.

The model shows the changes in age-specific death rates that accompany increases in life expectancy at birth. This distribution reveals a general pattern characterized by greater mortality in infancy, a minimum rate in the 5–14 year age group, and finally a progressive increase that reaches its peak in the group aged 65 and over. When life expectancy is low, all the death rates are high, especially among the youngest and oldest. As life expectancy increases, all ages experience a reduction in mortality, but the greatest gains are observed in children under 5. In this age group, when life expectancy rises from 50 to 75 years, the risk of dying is reduced from 40.8 to only 3.9

per 1000. This represents a substantial reduction—90%. In other words, of ten children who died before their fifth birthday when life expectancy at birth was 50 years, only one dies when life expectancy reaches 75. The under-5 age group is where the greatest absolute and relative reductions take place, but all the remaining age groups also show sizable reductions, with different implications depending on their level of mortality. Thus, the group aged 5–14 also experiences a reduction of approximately 90%; the 15–39 year-old group, 80%; the 40–64 year-old group, 64%; and the elderly (65 and older), 34%. It is notable that this last age group is the one which, after the first (children under 5), shows the greatest absolute reduction, since the rate declines from 91 to 60 per 1000 (Table 1 and Figure 1).

Table 1. Mortality rates by age, according to life expectancy at birth, Cuba-Costa Rica model.

Life expectancy at birth	Mortality rates by age (per 1,000)				
	0–4	5–14	15–39	40–64	65 and over
50	40.8	2.8	5.5	16.9	91.0
55	33.5	2.2	4.3	14.2	84.0
60	26.2	1.6	3.2	11.5	77.1
65	18.5	1.0	2.2	9.2	72.1
70	10.6	0.6	1.6	7.6	66.3
75	3.9	0.3	1.1	6.1	59.7

Source: CELADE, 1989.

The reduction of mortality in the elderly population implies that survival at 65 years increases from 11 to 17 years, or a total of 6 years. On the other hand, a reduction in mortality before 65 years (between the models based on 50 and 75 years of life expectancy at birth) means that almost twice as many persons as before will live to the age of 65. This aging of the population is a critical factor in all the countries of the Region. It varies in relative importance, but it must be reckoned with as an irreversible trend. It means that plans have to be made to provide health care to older age groups, without neglecting the rest of the population. In the United States of America the estimated populations under 18 and over 65 represented 25.8% and 12.7%, respectively, of the total population in 1990. By the year 2030 those percentages will be practically equal: 21.7% and 20.7%. In Uruguay it is predicted that by 2025 the percentages of females under 15 and over 65 will be 20% and 16%, respectively.

The speed of demographic change in Latin America becomes evident when one compares the values for proportional mortality by age with the different values for life expectancy. This is

Figure 1. Mortality from broad groups of causes in children under five years of age, according to life expectancy at birth.

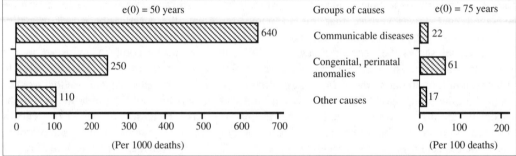

especially marked in children under 5, despite the fact that in this group proportional mortality continues to be much higher than the levels in the developed countries, with a life expectancy at birth of 75 years due to the age distribution of the population. Thus Costa Rica, whose infant mortality is one of the lowest rates in the Region but where 15% of total deaths occur before the fifth birthday, stands in contrast to Canada, where deaths in this age group are below 2%. An analogous but inverse situation occurs with proportional mortality in the group aged 65 and over.

The factors that are most involved in accounting for the increase in life expectancy at birth have to do with the communicable diseases, especially the reduction in deaths from infectious intestinal and respiratory diseases. It is estimated that between 1965 and 1990 there were more than 6 million deaths in Latin America and the Caribbean caused by intestinal infections (diarrhea), 80% of which occurred in children under 5. This cause alone accounted for 9% of total mortality. It can be estimated that the annual average of deaths due to diarrhea was more than 130 000 in the five-year period 1985-1990, a figure which underscores the problem's persistence.

For children under 5 we have seen that the reduction in mortality was 90%, so that if 1000 died previously, now only 100 die. The distribution of these deaths by major groups of causes is shown in Figure 1. The changes in the distribution of causes also are given for the other age groups; the overall changes can be evaluated based on an analysis of proportional mortality by ages. Previously, almost half of all deaths occurred before 5 years of age and now almost 60% occur after age 65 (Figure 2).

Analogous to the changes observed in the profile of mortality by age are the changes in terms of causes: for those whose life expectancy at birth was 50 years, almost two-thirds of the deaths were caused by communicable diseases and conditions originating in the perinatal period, whereas for those with a 75-year life expectancy a similar percentage is accounted for by malignant neoplasms, diseases of the circulatory system, and injury and poisoning.

There is cause for concern in the trend toward increasing death rates due to malignant neoplasms, especially in view of the fact that effective preventive measures now exist for several of these tumors. Death rates due to lung cancer are on the increase in almost all the countries. They are much higher in Argentina, Canada, Cuba, the United States, and Uruguay than in the remaining countries, and they are higher among males. Death rates in both sexes for malignant stomach tumors are unusually high in Barbados, Chile, Costa Rica, Ecuador, and Venezuela. The highest mortality rates for cervical tumors are concentrated in some of the countries of the English-speaking Caribbean, and the increase is most marked at younger ages, beginning at age 35. The highest mortality rates for malignant tumors of the breast are recorded in Argentina, Barbados, Canada, the United States, and Uruguay, and the rates rise with increasing age, being most marked after age 35.

Diseases of the circulatory system have come to constitute the most important cause of death in the countries with an older age distribution, where they account for more than one-third and in some of the cases more than two-fifths of the total deaths from defined causes. This is true despite the fact that the value of the rates tends to decline—although not before mortality from ischemic heart disease took on epidemic proportions, predominantly among males and especially in the group aged 45-54.

In the countries that have succeeded in reducing their death rates, especially those that have already achieved a life expectancy at birth of 70 years or more, accidents and acts of violence are the leading causes of death among schoolchildren and young adults, with a definite male predominance in the latter case. Prevention of this group of causes is another great challenge for public health.

The increase in proportional mortality from a specific cause in a specific age group does not necessarily imply that in that age group the specific death rate from that cause has increased; the

Figure 2. Proportional mortality according to life expectancy at birth.

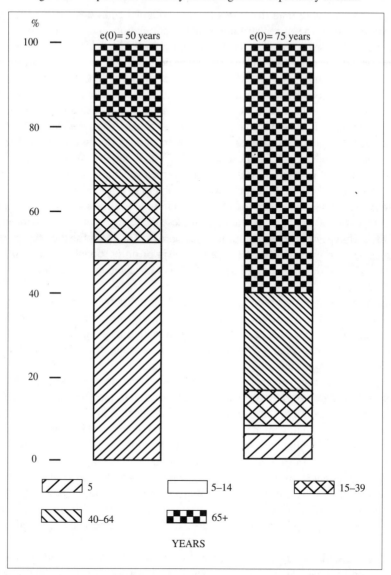

rate may have decreased, but reductions in the rates for other causes in that age group may have been even greater. Up to 40 years of age, there was a real reduction in the rates from all causes; between ages 40 and 64 the reduction also was sizable, with one important exception: malignant neoplasms present a deteriorating rate that continues up to the end of life. As has been shown, another important group of causes, diseases of the circulatory system, is increasingly the most important cause of death despite the fact that there have been improvements in the rates, especially in the groups aged 40 and older.

There are some peculiarities linked to the physical environment. For example, for a 50-year life expectancy at birth in those countries with more temperate climates, deaths due to respiratory diseases are greater than those from intestinal infections, whereas in countries with a tropical climate the reverse is true. On the other hand, of the 185 000 deaths registered in Canada (1987), 1100 were due to infectious and parasitic diseases (0.6% of the total) and only 38 were due to infectious intestinal diseases, none of which occurred in infants under 1 year. By contrast, of the 811 000 deaths registered in Brazil (1986), 51 500 were due to infectious and parasitic diseases (6.4% of the total), or 10 times more, but there also were 24 200 deaths from infectious intestinal diseases, 18 000 of which occurred in infants under 1 year old. Death rates due to pneumonia are only slightly higher in Mexico than in Canada (1987), but while in the latter country only 25 of the 5800 deaths from that cause occurred in the first year of life (0.4%), in Mexico the proportion was 8700 out of 20 500 (42.4%). Therefore, there is a contrast that is not reflected in the rate: in Canada, pneumonia is a cause of death at older ages and in Mexico at younger ones.

The figures show overall declining trends in the maternal mortality rates. Complications of pregnancy, delivery, and the puerperium play an important role as a cause of death for women in all or some of the subgroups within the 15–44 age range. The figures should be interpreted with caution, however, given the varying degrees of underestimation due to underregistration or assignment to other causes, which happens much more often in those countries where the problem is most serious. For maternal mortality, underregistrations have been estimated to exceed 50%. The available data for recent years in countries of the Region reveal significant variations: high values of around 25 maternal deaths per 10 000 live births for Bolivia, Haiti, Honduras, and Peru, compared with a low of 0.6 for Canada.

Migration

In addition to fertility and mortality, international migration is the other demographic component that affects the growth and distribution of the population by sex and age. It is highly dependent on the combination of the socioeconomic and political factors that prevail at any given time. Although in some cases migration significantly affects the age distribution of the population, especially in small countries, it does not become a fundamental factor in the aging process over the long term.

This is the most difficult demographic variable to measure, since records of population movements across national borders are usually deficient or nonexistent. To this is added so-called illegal migration, a trend apparently accentuated in the last decades; obviously, its inherently clandestine nature limits efforts to measure it.

An analysis of the 1970 and 1980 censuses shows an overall increase in mobility throughout the Hemisphere, as well as a substantial presence of Latin Americans and Caribbean nationals in the United States of America and Canada. Preliminary data from the United States Census estimates an increase of 8 million in the number of Latin Americans between 1980 and 1990, representing growth on the order of 60%. In addition, there is a steady decline in European migration to the Latin American countries.

Particularly notable in Central America are the movements linked to political conflicts and wars, which produce internal population displacements along with a significant number of refugees. To these are added persons who have been returned and repatriated under the provisions of the Esquipulas peace plan.

A persistent characteristic of the demographic situation in the English-speaking Caribbean countries is the high incidence of international migration. Although there are certain variations among the countries, there is unquestionably a sustained migratory flow directed largely toward North America and Western Europe.

Special attention is given to health problems in the receiving countries, which face an increased demand for care due to the arrival of new population groups that are often in precarious socioeconomic conditions. The cases that present the greatest problems are those involving short-distance cross-border migrations, often linked to harvesting, and those involving populations seeking refuge from the conflicts in the Central American subregion.

The short-distance movement across borders presents certain problems that the health sector must deal with: the need to provide health care to a population that usually works in an illegal situation and in very precarious and disadvantaged social conditions, as well as the problem of disease transmission across borders. Moreover, evidence points to a likely increase in this type of movement in the coming years as a result of efforts by the countries to create areas of increased economic integration.

In recent years, one of the significant problems for the health sector has been the populations migrating to other countries as political refugees or because they are fleeing violence. Figures from several sources suggest that between 7% and 10% of the Central American population has had to emigrate, in most cases as undocumented migrants to foreign countries or as persons displaced to another region within their own country, with a smaller proportion as recognized refugees or repatriated persons. This involves a total of around 2 million persons who have been abruptly expelled from their countries and who require immediate assistance in order to meet all types of social needs. The problem worsened because of the fact that only a minority are accorded the benefits of the United Nations High Commission for Refugees (UNHCR).

Urbanization and the environment

As a rule, both fertility and mortality are usually lowest in urban areas, and in most of the developing countries the health systems offer greater coverage in these areas, given the scarcity of resources and the more or less generalized development model that favors the concentration of resources in those areas where economic investment and productive, commercial, cultural, and political activities are concentrated as well.

The urbanization process also has produced overall inequities between the urban and rural areas in terms of economic, labor, and social affairs, and in the health sector in particular, creating large differentials in mortality, fertility, and morbidity between the urban and rural populations. This situation prevails in most of the Region's countries.

Differences occur not only between urban and rural areas but also among urban nuclei, with goods and services tending to concentrate in a few centers to the detriment of the rest, so that the situation of the latter is sometimes very similar to that of the rural areas. Finally, although the provision of goods and services—including those related to health—is greater in the large urban centers, the entire population does not necessarily have equal access to them, with large discrepancies between the socioeconomic strata that make up the population.

As a result of the marked difference in the dynamism of the urban and rural populations, the Region of the Americas as a whole ceased to have a predominantly rural population by the beginning of the 1950s. However, Latin America did not lose its rural predominance until the 1960s, and the Caribbean area, until the 1970s. Thus, in 1990, 28% of the population of the Americas was living in so-called rural areas, with estimates that this segment will fall to one-fourth of the total population by the year 2000.

It is already well known that the Region's rural population shows a low growth rate, going from 0.8% average annual growth in the 1950s to 0.5% in the five-year period 1985–1990, with the decline expected to continue. The lower growth rate for the rural population that is observed in most of the countries of the Americas is more a reflection of migration to urban areas than of a decline in the natural growth rate. The causes of these migrations in the developing countries are principally linked to the search for better opportunities for employment, education, and health, and, ultimately, the search for a better life.

On the other hand, it is estimated that in 1990, 73% of the population of the Americas was living in urban areas, with predictions that by the year 2000, 76 of every 100 persons will live in these areas. Although North America outpaces Latin America in degree of urbanization, by the year 2000 the two subregions will show similar proportions. The Caribbean, for its part, has a lower level of urbanization (60% in 1990 and an expected 66% by the year 2000), but even so, the area has ceased to have a rural predominance. From 475 million in 1985, the urban population in the Region of the Americas increased by 54 million in the five-year period 1985–1990—in contrast with the rural population, which increased by 5 million—and it is predicted to reach 626 million by the year 2000.

It should be noted, however, that due to the different rate of growth of this population in the subregions, in North America the urban population by the year 2000 will be 8% more than in 1990, whereas in Latin America and the Caribbean it will be 28% more, posing a serious challenge to meet basic needs in urban areas.

The process of urban concentration analyzed above has led to rising prices for urban land, along with land speculation, which has prevented a great many people from being able to secure decent housing in a healthy environment. Moreover, housing construction policies are based on lending systems that exclude those sectors of the population that are below the poverty line. The social housing policies that have been implemented in many of the Latin American countries have tended to apply to small-scale projects, encouraging and, at times, forcing the poorer sectors to move to peripheral neighborhoods or to crowd into shantytowns in the city's core.

In inner-city districts the population density is such that sometimes entire families occupy single rooms of what used to be large residential houses that are now rented by rooms, without any increase in the number of bathrooms. The poor condition of their surroundings is compounded by the inferior quality of the dwellings, which are typically constructed of flimsy or salvaged materials (clay, cardboard, straw) and in most cases are but one small room with virtually no ventilation.

This type of settlement, along with the displacement of the more economically comfortable sectors to suburban areas, has resulted in ecological deterioration in many cities of Latin America. Taking lands out of cultivation and eroding the urban perimeter (by felling trees and paving streets in high-altitude zones) impedes normal absorption of the rains, resulting in periodic floods.

The condition of the water, air, and wastes is indicative of the level of deterioration and pollution. The rate of water pollution is far worse in Latin America than in other regions of the world. It is estimated that less than 10% of the *municipios* in Latin America and the Caribbean treat wastewater adequately before discharging it into natural water bodies. In several of the countries, discharges from sewerage systems have contaminated rivers and other waterways—a situation that becomes even more dangerous when these waters are used to irrigate fields and vegetable gardens. The cholera cases that recently appeared in Chile's central valley originated precisely in this way.

Urban air pollution is the result of industrial activity, automobiles, electric power generation, and service industries. In the countries of Latin America and the Caribbean where tetraethyl lead is added to gasoline, the air is also contaminated with fine lead particles. Almost all the large cities in Latin America have problems with air quality, particularly Caracas, Mexico City, Lima, Rio de Janeiro, Santiago, and São Paulo. The Region is increasing its participation in the worldwide problem of air pollution. According to data published by the World Resources Institute, of the total carbon monoxide produced by human activities, Latin America contributed 1% in 1950, 3% in 1965, and 4.7% in 1983. This problem is perpetuated by the population growth, especially in urban areas, which results in greater consumption of energy, more vehicles, and industrial growth.

The rapid increase in automobile traffic not only produces congestion and high rates of traffic accidents, but in many cases, because of inadequate vehicle maintenance and the geographical location of cities in valleys surrounded by mountains, it also produces high levels of "smog." In 1984, the gasolines used in the Region contained the highest levels of lead in the world, ranging from 0.64 to 0.84 g/l, in comparison with, for example, Europe, where levels ranged from 0.15 to 0.40 g/l for the same year.

With the growth of the cities there has been a considerable increase in industrial and household waste, and in many cities the urban collection systems can no longer cope. In marginal communities this service is often limited, sporadic, or nonexistent, exacerbating already unhealthy conditions. Uncovered refuse dumps lie in open fields near marginal human settlements, attracting and favoring the breeding of animals that transmit diseases and release large quantities of methane gas. In many cities of Latin America, scavenging from refuse is a source of income for the very poorest population.

The coverage with refuse services reaches 81.7% of the population in Latin America. It is estimated that the quantity of solid wastes generated in 1988 by 300 million urban inhabitants of Latin America reached 225 000 tons per day. This refuse, which used to be predominantly organic and easily biodegradable, now includes a variety of materials with more inorganic substances and even toxic contaminants.

Factories and industries that were originally on the outskirts of the cities are now inside the urban perimeter. Some of them discharge highly toxic residues and wastes such as mercury, lead, magnesium, chromium, and even radioactive materials, which are destroying the organic components of the environment. In addition, there are other installations such as electric power plants, oil refineries, and hospitals that generate large amounts of toxic waste.

In the Americas there are few installations for recycling or properly disposing of hazardous waste. The current practice of "dumping" hazardous and nonhazardous waste should be reviewed and the necessary measures must be taken to deal with the situation at both the national and the international levels.

Employment

In the mid-1970s the major labor problem in the countries of Latin America and the Caribbean was not unemployment, but underemployment. Studies of the decade estimated that only one-fifth of the underutilization of labor in Latin America was due to open unemployment. In the urban areas the rate of open unemployment in Latin America and the Caribbean for 13 of the countries averaged 7%. In 1980, open unemployment reached an average of 8% in a group of 20 countries. In general, it was in the more urbanized countries that the rate of open unemployment fell, while it increased in the predominantly rural countries that are in the process of urbanization. As urbanization advanced in the more rural countries, it appeared to trigger increases in open unemployment. However, this is not the only factor that appears as a cause of this trend, since eminently urban countries, such as Chile and Peru, also saw increases. When the crisis of the 1980s began, the rate of urban open unemployment in Latin America and the Caribbean increased considerably, reaching an average of 11% in 1985.

To the increases in unemployment and underemployment are added the decline in real wages in several of the Latin American countries and the increase in poverty and indigence within their cities. One of the population's main ways of dealing with this drop has been to put more members of the family to work, with women and teenagers engaging in marginal occupations. As a result, they have to work longer hours to maintain their standard of living, or simply to meet minimum needs. Another response has involved sharing living quarters.

Morbidity

It is estimated that in the Region of the Americas the population at risk of contracting malaria increased from 143.6 million (30% of the total) in 1960 to 280.7 million in 1988 (39% of the total). Malaria transmission is concentrated in areas where the human population comes into close contact with the population of anopheline vectors for various sociopolitical, economic, and cultural reasons.

Generally speaking, the problem of malaria is found mainly in the territories in the area of the Great Amazon Basin—in Brazil, Bolivia, Colombia, Ecuador, French Guiana, Guyana, Peru, Suriname, and Venezuela —which have similar geographic and ecological characteristics. There are also shared risk factors linked to the development of the countries' social and economic infrastructure, such as migration and land settlements related to the expansion of the agricultural border, the building of roads, and projects involving agriculture, livestock, mining, and urban development.

The number of malaria cases reported by the countries increased steadily during 1985–1988. From a figure of 910 917 cases in 1985, the number climbed to more than one million in the next few years—1 018 864 in 1987 and 1 100 330 in 1988. The reporting of these cases corresponds to the number diagnosed by microscopic examinations carried out by the malaria control programs, based on an average of 9.8 million blood samples taken annually between 1985 and 1988. The percentage of blood samples with plasmodia increased from 9.6% in 1985 to 11.4% in 1988. Morbidity per 100 000 population in the malarious areas increased from 350.9 in 1965 to 391.9 in 1988.

Jungle yellow fever continues to affect the Americas, especially in four countries: Bolivia, Brazil, Colombia, and Peru. Cases of the disease also occasionally were reported in Ecuador, Trinidad and Tobago, and Venezuela. There have been no registered cases of urban yellow fever in South America since 1942, and the last outbreak of yellow fever in a large city occurred in Rio de Janeiro in 1928 and 1929.

The danger of the disease's urbanization constitutes a real threat, given the increase and spread of *Aedes aegypti* populations in urban centers, some of which are located near enzootic areas of yellow fever. This situation may be potentially aggravated by the recent introduction into Brazil of *Aedes albopictus*, a vector whose particular characteristics could potentially bridge the jungle and urban cycles of the disease.

During 1985–1988, 754 cases were reported in five countries of the Region. This number represents an increase of 238 cases (46.1%) compared to the previous four-year period. Approximately 85% of the cases were fatal. The official figures probably underestimate the magnitude of the problem, since it is mostly the fatal cases that are registered.

Circulation of the dengue virus in the Americas during the decade took the form of major epidemics. To date only serotypes 1, 2, and 4 have been isolated from the autochthonous cases occurring in the Americas during the 1980s. One of the major events of the decade was the epidemic of hemorrhagic dengue caused by dengue 2 that occurred in Cuba in 1981. Dengue 4 has become endemic in the Region, after causing a series of outbreaks in the Caribbean, Central America, Mexico, and northern South America, especially during 1981–1983. The disease associated with dengue 4 has been generally mild and self-limiting. After 1981, every year (except 1983) saw reports of confirmed or suspected cases of dengue hemorrhagic fever in both children and adults.

The transmission of the wild poliovirus appears on the verge of being interrupted in the Western Hemisphere. Despite the analysis of thousands of fecal samples, only seventeen isolations of wild poliovirus were recovered in 1990, and four during the first six months of 1991. More than four years have elapsed since wild poliovirus was last isolated in the Southern Cone, and more than eight years since one was found in the English-speaking Caribbean. It has been more than three years since an autochthonous wild poliovirus was isolated in Central America, two years since one was isolated in Brazil, and five months since one was found in Mexico. The 17 wild viruses isolated in 1990 represent a reduction with respect to the 24 found in 1989.

Despite the general increase in vaccination coverage, outbreaks of measles continue to occur in several countries of the Region. This reflects the fact that, with the exception of Cuba, even the countries with high immunization coverage did not achieve the levels necessary to ensure the interruption of transmission.

The registration of information on diarrheal diseases in children is more deficient for morbidity than for mortality. Given that in a high percentage of cases no medical care is sought, there is no certainty about the real magnitude of the problem in any of the countries. However, it is possible to have an idea of the total number of diarrheal episodes in children under 5 based on the countries' estimates of annual incidence. For 1988 it may be estimated that there were an average of four diarrheal episodes per year in children under 5. This figure varies: values of five or more were estimated for the Dominican Republic, Guatemala, Haiti, Mexico, Peru, and Venezuela; values of between three and five, for Argentina, Bolivia, Brazil, Colombia, Costa Rica, Cuba, Ecuador, El Salvador, Honduras, and Panama; and values of under three, for Belize, Chile, Jamaica, Suriname, and Uruguay.

In 1990, studies on neonatal tetanus were conducted in 16 endemic countries of Latin America. The data indicate that 1,276, or 57%, of the known cases occurred in 5% (606) of the municipalities, where 10 million (11%) of the women of reproductive age in those countries live. In total regional figures, the cases affect 21% of the municipalities.

The chronic noncommunicable diseases, for the most part, are preceded by risk factors, sometimes common ones, that can be measured in the general population. In 1986, a Study on Individual and Population Risk Factors utilized a common methodology in limited areas of Latin American cities—Caracas (Venezuela), Ciudad Acuña and Piedras Negras (Mexico), Havana (Cuba), Porto Alegre (Brazil), and Santiago (Chile)—and found that the percentage of adults (15 years or older) exposed to hypertension, smoking, a sedentary lifestyle, and daily alcohol intake is high in comparison with the figures reported in the literature, although there are large differences between the values in the areas studied. There is a greater prevalence of smoking and daily alcohol consumption among males, but a higher prevalence of hypertension and sedentary lifestyle among females.

AIDS may well be the best example of the health impact of habits and customs, including sexual behavior and drug addiction. All 46 countries and territories of the Americas have reported cases of AIDS. Although the virus has been introduced in different countries at different times, once transmission is firmly established, the course of the epidemic has been similar in every country.

In the Region as a whole, it is estimated that approximately 2.5 million people are infected with HIV. Of these, between 1 million and 1.5 million live in North America, and approximately 750 000 to 1 million are located in Latin America and the Caribbean. The cumulative number of cases and deaths as of 31 October 1990 was 183 121 and 107 828, respectively. Eighty-three percent of the cases and 87% of the deaths have been in the United States.

Food and nutrition

In recent decades the food supply has increased considerably and nutritional status has improved. The world now feeds twice as many people as it did in 1950, and Latin America almost tripled its feeding capacity in the same period: from 160 million to 440 million. Indications of this quantitative improvement are the substantial reduction in infant mortality and the reduction in nutritional deficiencies as reflected in the size and weight of newborn infants. Food supplies are greater, and transportation, conservation, and distribution methods have improved.

Despite these advances, hunger and malnutrition continue to be problems at the regional level: in some countries of Latin America, per capita caloric intake has been lower in the last few years than it was at the beginning of the 1980s, and in 1983–1985 the food supply (apparent consumption) was 10% below minimum needs in several countries. In 1990, per capita grain production fell 16% with respect to 1981, with the annual level currently estimated at 210 kg per capita. This figure is worrisomely near the minimum of 180, below which long-term survival is impossible. The annual level in North America was 1324 kg per capita in 1990.

UNICEF estimates that there were 8 million undernourished children under 5 (more than two standard deviations below the desired level of weight-for-age) in Latin America and the Caribbean in 1990, representing 14% of the total population in that age group.

In several countries, vitamin A deficiency is a serious problem. Apparent consumption at mid-decade in Latin America and the Caribbean was 665 mcg, a level below that for Africa and one-half the value for the developed countries. Regarding iron and iodine levels, the situation is similar, although not quite as severe. In several of the countries, programs have been developed to provide supplementary feeding and improve the nutritional situation through iodization of salt; injections of iodized oil; education regarding food storage and consumption; distribution of ferrous sulfate; development of school and community vegetable gardens; and monitoring for the early detection of nutritional problems in pregnant women, women who have just given birth, and children.

The growth rate of food production decreased from 3.4% in 1970–1979 to 2.4% per year in 1980–1987. The high growth rates in 1985 and 1987 compensated for slower growth in 1980–1984. However, the importance of food exports in several of the countries led to less internal availability and, therefore, lower consumption. Not only did prices increase, but the population's food subsidy programs often were eliminated.

Education

In recent decades, there have been major advances in education. Illiteracy fell from 42% in 1950 to 15% in 1990 in Latin America and the Caribbean, with values about the same for both sexes, although in several countries illiteracy continues to be higher among women. The last few years have seen increased school enrollments, particularly at the middle and upper levels. In 1990 there were no sex differences in primary, secondary, and high-school enrollments, although at this last level, female attrition is greater and the career tracks favor males in those fields that lead to better jobs, especially jobs at decision-making levels.

The ongoing trend toward women's greater professionalization may bring about social structure changes in the medium and long term. This is especially true for careers related to health, where in several countries female enrollment already exceeds that of males. As a result of this trend, and despite attrition, in some years there have been more women graduating as physicians than men. This means that the educational trends among women have dual repercussions for the health of the population as a whole: on the one hand, a positive impact due to women's key role in determining the family's attitudes toward health, and on the other, steadily increasing labor participation by women as health workers (nurses, aides, and health professionals). In fact, it may well be that—although there have been no empirical studies in the Region to confirm it—the latter phenomenon will also benefit health, not in terms of demand (a more highly educated female population) but in terms of supply, as more women work and make decisions in the health sector.

Conclusions

Over the past decade, the Latin American and Caribbean countries have been affected by the most severe economic crisis since the 1930s. As a result, there has been an alarming increase in the rates of unemployment and internal inflation, along with a gradual deterioration in the supply of goods and services, especially in the public sector. The greatest obstacle to development continues to be the crisis of Latin American indebtedness: today, Latin America and the Caribbean are net exporters of capital to the industrialized countries. In the last five years (1986–1990), Latin American countries have sent US$130 billion abroad as payments on the accumulated external debt.

Consequently, the countries have had to adopt adjustment or reactivation economic policies that are characterized by a marked reduction in public spending for so-called "non-productive activities," such as health and education. The application of these measures has led to a reduction or stagnation in the amount of resources available for developing and operating the health services. This can be seen in the limitations on capital investment for basic sanitation and for the replacement, maintenance, and conservation of equipment and the physical plant. In addition, the situation affects the capacity to maintain an adequate level of recurrent expenditures, which has impeded normal program operations for dealing with prevalent problems and has restricted administrative development and personnel training in the sector. As a result, one of the most salient features in the countries of Latin America and the Caribbean, especially those of greater relative development—both because of the importance of health as an expenditure and because of the large share that health-related employment represents in the total work force—is the lack of regularly supplied information and permanent organization in the Ministries designed to meet the demands for data on economy, financing, and costs in the sector. This is an area that has received no consideration up to now.

At the same time, the economic crisis has adversely affected the well-being of vast sectors of the population. At present, nearly one-third of the population lives below the absolute poverty level. This poverty is distributed unequally within the individual countries, contributing to the increased disparities observed in the Region. In terms of coverage, of the 423 million inhabitants of Latin America and the Caribbean, some 130 million do not currently have permanent access to basic health services. Moreover, estimates of population growth indicate that during 1990–2000 there will be an additional 110 million inhabitants for whom adequate health care must be ensured. This represents the most important challenge for the health systems of the countries of the Region. It means that the services —which for the most part have so far been unable to serve the entire population with equity, effectiveness, and efficiency—must be reorganized and reoriented, not only in order to maintain their operations but also to close the current gap and respond to the health care needs of the new population.

In most of the reporting countries a deterioration can be seen in the efforts to implement a process for the surveillance and evaluation of the strategy of primary health care and health for all by the year 2000. No program, structure, or stable standards have been established for these activities. The data needed for monitoring and evaluation are obtained haphazardly, with serious problems of acquisition and without the involvement of the principal authorities in the sector's institutions. Save for Canada, Cuba, and the United States, which have clearly evaluated their targets and progress and have proposed new objectives, the remaining reports are more responses to a formal commitment to the Organization than an analysis and a reflection of what is happening. Among them are reports from a number of countries that have made substantial efforts: Haiti, Bolivia, the Bahamas, Belize, Honduras, Costa Rica, and Mexico. In the overall picture, however, the prospects are not encouraging with respect to the future possibilities for monitoring and evaluating primary health care and health for all by the year 2000.

The information on vaccination coverage is up-to-date in almost all the countries, reflecting the effort to eradicate wild poliovirus. In addition, data on coverage of the population with basic water supply and sanitation services are available in most of the countries, although there continue to be problems of consistency, continuity, and accuracy. However, reliable information on nutritional status, low birthweight, coverage with basic health care and maternal and child health services, family planning, and expenditures on health and local care is available in only a few countries. The data on referrals and back-referrals, mental and physical disabilities, oral health, and morbidity are practically nonexistent in most of the countries.

Once resources for neglected groups have been identified and obtained, the lack of focus and the transparency of the projects have been a critical factor, since it will present a major obstacle to studying their impact.

The obstacles to setting up a monitoring and evaluation process in the countries may be grouped under three main headings:

—those attributable to the lack of necessary human resources and infrastructure to collect and analyze the information adequately;
—the inferior quality of the data available due to underregistration, dispersion of sources, lack of timely delivery, and shortcomings in data processing; and
—limited contact within the health system between the management process and the information system for decision-making.

The national health policies and strategies in all the Region's countries are coherent and verbally consistent with the strategy of primary health care and health for all by the year 2000. The adaptation of these policies and strategies has been curtailed by the limits on financial, material, and human resources, and in some countries, by political and social instability. Health development in the Region is directed toward achieving greater efficiency in the use of available resources through restructuring the health systems—a process that includes decentralization, strengthening of local health systems, administrative reform, mobilization of local resources, and interinstitutional and intersectoral coordination. However, in many countries of Latin America and the Caribbean, long-term comprehensive strategies for the development of health and the overall socioeconomic situation are seen to be weak or entirely lacking, which makes it difficult to maintain the rate of improvement observed in the last 30 years.

Improved coordination among the institutions that make up the health sector in the countries of the Region is a goal shared by almost all. However, with few exceptions, this is reported to still be an incipient process, particularly with regard to coordination of the services provided by social security institutions and the Ministries of Health.

The reporting countries concur in stating that practically all the national sectors that participate in the overall development process have a direct or an indirect impact on the state of the population. Diverse institutional mechanisms have been established to ensure that the goals and activities of the different development sectors are coherent and mutually supportive, both in relation to overall development policy and among themselves. In several countries of the Region one of the goals in the effort to develop local health systems under a decentralized management scheme has been to encourage and facilitate the creation of operational mechanisms for joint programming and coordination among sectors at the local level. Other measures undertaken to improve this aspect of the primary health care strategy range from the formulation of constitutional mandates for coordination among sectors to the formal participation of health sector authorities in the administration of other institutions linked to health.

All the countries of the Region have manifested, as their declared policy, the need to support and promote community participation as an essential component of the primary health care strategy. In most cases, the community is involved in specific aspects of carrying out activities at the local level, especially through the mechanism of health collaborators or volunteers or by providing labor and funds for small local infrastructure projects. In some of the countries, mechanisms have been established for the participation of community organizations in the formulation, execution, and evaluation of policies and programs at the national level. In others, the Ministries of Health have created programs, offices, or departments responsible for promoting, coordinating, and standardizing community participation in health programs.

Since 1985, several countries have reviewed and modified the sector's institutional, organic, and functional framework with a view to opening the way for new management designs. The normative, regulatory, and controlling role of central levels in the Ministries or Secretariats of Health has been strengthened, and the executive functions and responsibilities of the peripheral arms of these institutions, or others involved in the delivery of services, have been increased. Others have had some success in defining the responsibilities and scope of the different institutions that make up the sector as a step preceding greater coordination and eventual intrasectoral integration. But these attempts at reforms have produced little result so far.

In some of the countries, steps have been taken to formulate and implement instruments and legal standards for the decentralized management of the health sector and of other public services. Moreover, many Ministries of Health in the Region have modified their technical and policy-making and administrative structures in accordance with the goal of decentralizing and facilitating the process of conducting and managing priority programs.

Of the reporting countries, few have a health manpower plan for meeting needs under the primary health care strategy, and few believe they have made progress since 1985 in improving equity in the distribution of human resources, while in fact some report a deterioration in equity. The principal reasons cited to account for this situation are the economic crisis, the restriction of financial resources, and the resistance of health personnel to being located in less developed areas. Several countries have instituted or strengthened programs for the training of professional and mid-level health personnel using an approach that integrates teaching and service. Many countries report having carried out recent curriculum revisions in professional training programs in order to incorporate more elements of public health and the primary health care strategy. In all the countries there are broad programs of continuing education for health personnel in specific aspects of the primary health care strategy; several have created inter-institutional commissions on health manpower as a way to improve coordination and planning in this field.

Few countries report the existence, even on paper or in incipient application, of a national policy for selecting and using health technology. In general, coordination of the selection and use of health technology is only weakly developed in most of the countries. With regard to the identification and formulation of national policies on health research, few countries have explicit guidelines in this area.

The orientations that have been defined correspond to priorities derived from the epidemiological profile and the level of development of the health services. The countries mention several factors that are impeding the effective preparation and application of policy on research and technology in the health field: the scarcity of financial resources, the lack of sufficient research personnel and infrastructure, the weakness of mechanisms of interinstitutional coordination, and the limited political will for promoting research as a development tool. The gap that is emerging between Latin America and the Caribbean, on the one hand, and the rest of the world (with the exception of Africa), on the other, with respect to the importance assigned and the resources being allocated for research and technology development is a critical negative element as far as the outlook for the future is concerned.

In terms of the trends observed in the Region in relation to coverage of the population by components of the primary health care strategy and to the overall health situation, the following stand out:

—Water and sanitation: moderate increase in coverage. There are major problems of access and quality, especially at the urban level, creating situations of serious risk, as witnessed by the cholera epidemic;

—Diseases covered by EPI: coverage with vaccines against polio, DPT, and measles has increased, reaching levels above 90% in many of the countries;

—Care provided for pregnant women, deliveries, and nursing infants: the information does not permit any firm conclusions, since only isolated and partial figures are available in most of the countries, although it is clear that in a majority of them the coverage is far from satisfactory, and for some countries the most recent data show a reduction in coverage;

—Coverage with primary health care: for this indicator the information is again insufficient to determine any trend for the Region;

—Mortality, birth rate, and life expectancy: these indicators show improvements, although to a lesser extent than in previous periods;

—Nutritional status and low birthweight: although only a very few countries have regular systems of nutritional surveillance, isolated data from surveys and special studies in most of the countries reveal the persistence of high levels of undernutrition in children, as well as low birthweight, in the Region.

In summary, there must be concerted efforts over the next few years to establish and strengthen not only the mechanisms for monitoring and follow-up of primary health care and health for all by the year 2000 strategy in the Region of the Americas but also the availability, coverage, and quality of the information. The current emphasis on the development of managerial and administrative schemes that are conducive to greater equity and efficiency in the utilization of resources should, in turn, stimulate consideration of the need to formulate and operationalize an information database for this purpose. Although some progress has been made, much remains to be done in the Region in this area, despite the fact that although the real degree of commitment that has been seen since the 1988 report does not leave much room for optimism in this regard.

Sources

Bolivia, "Encuesta Nacional de Demografía y Salud 1989, Instituto Nacional de Estadística/ Institute for Resource Development, 1990.

CELADE, "América Latina: Proyecciones de población, 1950–2025," 1990.

ECLAC, "Balance preliminar de la economía de América Latina y Centroamérica," 1990.

ECLAC, "Transformación productiva con equidad," CEPAL, 1990.

ECLAC/UNDP/UNFPA, "Magnitud de la pobreza en América Latina en los años ochenta."

Inter-American Development Bank, Economic and Social Progress in Latin America, 1990.

International Monetary Fund, Government Finance Statistics Yearbook, 1990.

National reports on Second Evaluation of HFA-2000.

PAHO, Directing Council, Report on the Monitoring of the Regional Strategies for Health for All by the Year 2000, 1988, CD33/22 Rev. 1.

PAHO, *Health Conditions in the Americas, 1990 Edition.* Scientific Publication 524.

PAHO, "Indicadores e información sobre las enfermedades diarreicas," 1990.

PAHO, Ninth Meeting of the Technical Advisory Group on Diseases Preventable by Vaccination, 1991.

PAHO, Regional Conference on Water Supply and Sanitation: Evaluation of the Drinking Water Supply and Sanitation Decade and Projections Towards the Year 2000, 1990.

UNDP, *Human Development Report, 1991.*

UNESCO, *Statistical Yearbook, 1990.*

UNICEF, *World Status of Children, 1991.*

United Nations, Report on the Social Situation in the World, 1989, New York, 1989.

World Bank, *World Development Report, 1990.*

World Bank, *World Development Report, 1991.*

World Bank, World Tables, 1991.

World Watch Institute, *State of the World, 1991.*

EVALUATION BY COUNTRY
AND OTHER POLITICAL UNITS

ARGENTINA

Demographic factors

The estimated population for 1990 was 32 322 000. In 1985–1990, the annual population growth was 1.27%. A total of 28.9% of the urban population and 36.2% of the rural population is under 15 years of age, and the population aged 60 years old and older represents 13.5% of the urban population and 10.7% of the rural. The urban population accounts for 85.9% of the total. The birthrate for 1985–1990 was estimated at 21.4 per 1000 inhabitants, and the fertility rate, at 3.0 children per woman.

Socioeconomic factors

The per capita GDP in 1990 was US$2260, and inflation for 1980–1989 was 334.8% per year. In 1990, it was estimated that urban unemployment was 7.4% and that 38.6% of households were poor. Illiteracy is estimated at 4.7%.

Health indicators

Total mortality for 1985–1990 was estimated at 8.6 per 1000 inhabitants, and was recorded as 8.0 per 1000 in 1987. Infant mortality reported in 1987 was 26.6 per 1000 live births; mortality from 1 to 4 years, 1.0 per 1000 children in that age group; and maternal mortality, 4.9 per 10 000 live births.

Life expectancy for 1985–1990 was estimated at 70.6 years.

The leading causes of death are diseases of the heart and malignant neoplasms, followed by infectious diseases.

No national figure is available for the proportion of children with birthweight under 2500 grams. A study carried out throughout the country in 1985 on a sample of 5600 public-school children in the first to third grades—excluding the capital city of Buenos Aires—revealed that 10% of the studied children aged 6 to 10 years old showed growth retardation.

Health care system

The health services system comprises the national Government, the 24 provincial governments, municipalities, social security institutions, the Armed Forces, and private hospitals and physicians. The system includes the public, social welfare, and private sectors.

The current health policy aims at improving the procurement and rational use of resources by the Ministry of Health and Social Action and the provincial ministries of health, as a way to promote decentralization and bring about political changes that will, in turn, lead to the implementation of structural change and the resolution of emergency situations. To this end, the development of intersectoral health programs and the design of appropriate planning methodologies for their formulation, management, and evaluation have been proposed.

In 1988, the National Health Insurance Law was passed, along with the new Social Welfare Law that is designed to extend coverage to self-employed workers and to all those in the country who have no coverage.

That same year, a process of federalization and decentralization of the health services was initiated; more than one-third of the jurisdictions have participated at different degrees of development.

Information systems have operated irregularly, which has hampered decision-making.

Spending on health represents 8.2% of the GDP; in 1985, 22.7% of health financing came from the public sector; 39.2%, from the social welfare sector; and 38.1%, from the private sector.

Argentina has 3186 hospitals and 147 000 beds, or approximately 5 beds per 1000 population; 31% of the beds are in private institutions.

Sophisticated, high-technology equipment is concentrated largely in private health establishments in the large cities. By 1988, there were 128 CAT scanners in the country, up from only 45 in 1985.

In 1985, the country had approximately 30 physicians, 7 dentists, 10 pharmacists, 3 biochemists, 8 psychologists, 5 nurses, 8 nursing auxiliaries, 4 physical therapists, and 1 midwife per 10 000 population.

Primary care

Primary care is mainly provided through 6456 outpatient facilities located throughout the country; 30% of them are in the Federal Capital and the Province of Buenos Aires. It has been acknowledged that there are some limitations in the resolution capacity of the secondary support network for these services. In order to improve primary care services, some provinces have initiated residences in general and/or family medicine.

In 1987, 96% of pregnant women received care provided by trained personnel, and 72% had been seen before the end of the first trimester of pregnancy; 94.5% of deliveries were in institutions, and 95.4% were attended by trained personnel.

Contraceptive methods are used by 43% of women with children under 4 years of age.

Immunization coverage in 1990 was 99% for BCG, 85% for DPT, 89% for polio vaccine, and 95% for measles vaccine. In 1988, 64.27% of the population had drinking water services (73.05% of the urban population and 16.87% of the rural), and 88.95% of the population had adequate excreta disposal systems (100% in urban areas and 29.27% in rural areas).

International cooperation for several projects is being provided both directly by other countries and by international agencies. Cooperation agreements have been signed with neighboring countries for the solution of common problems.

BAHAMAS

Demographic factors

The estimated population in 1990 was 255 000, 80% of which lives on two of the islands, New Providence and Grand Bahama. The annual growth rate was estimated at 1.82% for 1985–1990. The population under 15 years of age represents 32.2% of the total. The birthrate for 1985–1990 was 20.7 per 1000 population, and the fertility rate, 2.17 children per woman.

Socioeconomic factors

The per capita GDP in 1989 was US$11 370. The illiteracy rate is estimated at 4.8%, and the unemployment rate in 1988 was estimated at 11%.

Health indicators

The mortality rate was 5.4 per 1000 population in 1988; infant mortality, 21.4 per 1000 live births; maternal mortality, 2 per 10 000 live births; and mortality in children aged 1–4, 0.91 per 1000 children in that age group.

Life expectancy at birth was estimated at 71.1 years for 1985–1990.

The leading causes of death are chronic diseases, mainly diseases of the heart, followed by malignant neoplasms and accidents. Pneumonia is the only infectious disease that appeared among the 10 leading causes of death in 1988.

The percentage of children with birthweight under 2500 grams was 7.83%, according to 1989 hospital records. However, a nutrition survey carried out in 1988–1989 showed low birthweight in 14.37% of newborns, and revealed that 2.2% of children under 1 year of age and 8.18% of children from 1 to 4 years of age were undernourished (based on weight-for-age).

Health care system

The health care system includes both a public and private sector. There are three public hospitals (one specialized in geriatric psychiatry) with 1100 beds, and two private, in addition to 45 public clinics with a total of 75 beds and 75 public clinics without beds. The country's insular geography has led to serious problems with the delivery of health care services, which, coupled with the lack of personnel trained in data processing and analysis, the large volume of data, and the lack of computerized data management systems, has made it difficult to exercise adequate surveillance in the islands.

In 1990, the Bahamas had 13.03 physicians, 1.70 dentists, 2.61 pharmacists, 24.1 registered nurses, 18.44 clinically-trained nurses, and 14.61 nursing auxiliaries per 10 000 population.

An automated system has been initiated at the central level for the primary health care reporting system. Similarly, an attempt has been made to improve the flow of information from the various islands through the installation of telephones and the use of first-class mail.

New primary health care centers have been put into operation, and primary health care services are now being provided in all clinics that did not offer it previously.

In 1989, the Dental Health Law was enacted and the Dental Council was established. Dental services are presently being expanded, and personnel is being trained in this area.

Education for family life was approved for inclusion in the school curriculum.

Management of the country's water resources, previously shared, has now been placed under a single administration.

Primary care

Although no official document prescribes a national strategy and plan of action, many activities are being carried out and priority health care areas have been identified. These include reducing child mortality, extending primary care, and further emphasizing child health. Recently, a Planning Committee was established in the Ministry of Health in conjunction with the Health Project for the Bahamas, and efforts have been made to set up a Planning Unit in the Ministry.

Community participation has focused more on supporting programs than on planning. Many groups are working on specific problems such as AIDS, drugs, and diabetes.

A National Health Insurance Plan is being prepared with the participation of numerous individuals from the community.

The official budget for health care represents 3.47% of the GDP. It is estimated that 99% of the entire population has easy access to health services, that a similar percentage of pregnant women receive prenatal care, and that 99% of deliveries are attended by trained personnel.

In 1989, immunization coverage for infants under 1 year of age was 86% for DPT and 82% for polio vaccine; the MMR (measles, mumps, and rubella) vaccine was administered to 87% of children 1 year of age. Of the pregnant women who sought public prenatal care services (approximately 80% of all pregnant women), coverage with tetanus toxoid was 75% for New Providence, 54.7% for Grand Bahama, and 48.1 for the Family Islands.

In 1988, 99.59% of the population had drinking water services (99.26% in urban areas and 100% in rural areas). According to the 1980 census, only 2.2% of the population lacked an adequate excreta disposal system (0.7% in New Providence and 0.1% in Grand Bahama); recent estimates indicate that this proportion remains unchanged.

BELIZE

Demographic factors

The population of Belize in 1990 was estimated at 189 000, and the annual growth rate for 1985–1990 was 2.60%. According to the 1980 census, 45% of the population is under 15 years of age; 52.7% of the population resides in urban areas. The birthrate recorded in 1989 was 37.2 per 1000 population, and the fertility rate was estimated at 5.2 children per woman.

Socioeconomic factors

In 1989 the per capita GDP was US$1720. In 1980, illiteracy was 5%.

Health indicators

In 1989, the total mortality was 4.2 per 1000 population; infant mortality, 19.4 per 1000 live births; maternal mortality, 0.36 per 10 000 live births; and mortality in children aged 1–4 years, 1.5 per 1000.

Life expectancy at birth in 1990 was estimated at 70.8 years.

In 1989, 12.7% of newborns weighed less than 2500 grams.

The leading causes of death in 1989 for all age groups were: other diseases of the respiratory system; diseases of pulmonary circulation and other forms of heart disease; certain conditions originating in the perinatal period; cerebrovascular disease; and endocrine and metabolic diseases and immunity disorders. In children under 1 year of age the most important causes of mortality were certain conditions originating in the perinatal period, other diseases of the respiratory system, congenital anomalies and nutritional deficiencies. For the same year, the most important reasons for hospitalization were normal delivery, direct obstetric causes, other diseases of the respiratory system, diseases of other parts of the digestive system, abortion, and intestinal infectious diseases.

Health care system

The Government of Belize recognizes health as a basic right and a fundamental condition for development, and it has therefore committed itself to providing health services for all citizens by means of community participation and intersec-toral coordination. The country's health policy is guided by the principles of democracy, integrity, education, participation, and accessibility. The main components of the policy are accessibility to the health services, health promotion, intersectoral coordination, and community participation.

The health plan identifies as priority groups mothers and children under 5 years of age, low-income groups, the disabled, the elderly, and those who live in underserved areas. Priority also is assigned to the prevention and treatment of highly prevalent diseases and conditions and to the training of human resources. The development of infrastructure at the district level and the construction of a hospital for tertiary care in the capital city are being emphasized.

Future actions include decentralization and deconcentration, the strengthening of administrative and managerial capacity, the development of information systems, the reinforcement of inter-sectoral ties, and the focusing on organization and policy matters.

In Belize, information is collected at all levels of the health system; this information is used largely for administrative purposes and, to a lesser degree, for planning, management, and decision-making.

Although no national information policy exists as such, certain priority areas have been defined, including nutrition.

In 1990, the country had 1 general hospital, 6 district hospitals and 32 health centers (9 urban and 23 rural), and a total of 300 beds (2.12 per 1000 population).

In the same year, there were 6.6 physicians, 0.7 dentists, 0.1 pharmacists, 9.0 nurses, 11.9 practical nurses, 2.0 nursing auxiliaries, and 1.0 midwives per 10 000 population. There are no significant differences in their distribution, although there is a greater concentration in the capital city, because of the presence of the hospital.

In 1989, spending on health represented 2.2% of the GDP, (9.5% of national public spending); 21.7% went to local services and 14.5% to primary care.

Primary care

The Ministry of Health is endeavoring to develop primary care through activities such as the preparation of a manual on primary care and the expansion of health care infrastructure.

Intersectoral coordination has only had limited development at the national level. Varying degrees of coordination and collaboration exist at the local level.

Community participation was initiated at the beginning of the 1980s with the development of town health committees and district health groups. The former are composed of people elected by the community who share a common interest in community health; the latter is made up of people from the district and government employees who work at that level.

Belize receives a significant amount of funding for its health programs from international agencies.

In 1989, 100% of the urban population and 95% of the rural population had access to health services; 91.5% of pregnant women, 94.8% of infants, and 82.7% of deliveries were attended by trained personnel. In 1990 the percentage of deliveries attended by trained personnel rose to 86.9%.

In 1989, 10.3% of the women of childbearing age were using contraceptive methods, and 39.4% of pregnant women received tetanus toxoid. Immunization coverage in children under 1 year of age in 1990 was 80% for BCG, 84% for DPT, 80% for polio vaccine, and 81% for measles vaccine.

In 1990, 95% of the urban population, 65% of the rural population, and 80% of the combined populations were supplied with drinking water services; 60%, 16%, and 43%, respectively, had adequate excreta disposal systems.

BOLIVIA

Demographic factors

In 1990, Bolivia had an estimated population of 7 171 000. The annual growth for 1985–1990 was 2.46%. Forty-nine percent of the total population in 1988 was rural; 44% of the population is under 15 years of age. The birthrate for 1985–1990 was estimated at 37.46 per 1000 population, and the fertility rate, at 5.0 children per woman.

Socioeconomic factors

The per capita GDP in 1989 was US$620. Inflation for 1980–1989 was 391.3% annually. Illiteracy is 22.5%, and urban unemployment was 9.5% in 1990.

Health indicators

The total estimated mortality for 1985–1990 was 10.6 per 1000 population, and infant mortality for the same period was 98 per 1000 live births per year (according to the 1989 National Demographic and Health Survey, infant mortality for that year was 96 per 1000). Maternal mortality in 1988 was 24.7 per 10 000 live births.

Life expectancy at birth for 1985–1990 was estimated at 58.9 years.

Mortality is underreported, and it is estimated that only 20% of deaths are recorded. The leading causes of death reported are infectious and parasitic diseases, primarily intestinal infections; tuberculosis; and other diseases preventable by vaccination.

In 1988, 9.26% of live born children had a birthweight lower than 2500 grams. It was reported that 11.1% of children under 5 years of age had weight-for-age deficits.

Health care system

The health sector is made up of three subsectors: the public sector (represented by the Ministry of Social Welfare and Public Health), which is estimated to cover 48% of the population; the social security system, with a coverage of 22%; and the private sector, to which it is estimated 10% of the population has access.

Regionalization began in 1985. Currently the public services include the central level, represented by the Ministry; the regional level, made up of health units; and the local level, comprising 94 health districts and 440 health areas.

The Government of Bolivia has assigned priority to education and health within the social sector. Health policy is cast within the context of the development process. Within the overall framework of the State's modernization, improvement of the quality of life, and reduction of the risks of disease and death in the most vulnerable population groups, priority is being assigned to activities aimed at mothers, children, workers, and environmental sanitation. For 1983–1993, the health policy has pursued three basic lines of action: implementation of the National Plan for Child Survival and Development and Maternal Health, the decentralization of the health services, and the promotion of grass-roots management.

The Plan of Action includes the following operational programs: comprehensive care for children under 5 years of age; care for schoolchildren and adolescents; comprehensive care for women of childbearing age; comprehensive care for the environment; epidemiological surveillance and control; and institutional strengthening.

In 1988, spending on health represented 2.2% of the GDP; of this amount the Ministry accounted for 0.9% and the social security system for 1.3%.

In 1991, the Bolivian public sector had 35 hospitals and 136 primary care centers in urban areas and 120 hospitals and 1058 primary health care centers in rural areas; it also had 110 private hospitals. The total number of beds was 9500.

In 1990, there were 5.09 physicians, 0.36 dentists, 2.40 nurses, 5.75 nursing auxiliaries, 0.21 social workers, and 0.20 nutritionists per 10 000 population. There is a high concentration of professionals at the secondary and tertiary care levels. In-service, continuing education programs have been established for health personnel.

Primary care

Primary care is provided at the district level, and special emphasis has been placed on 17 districts. In well-organized districts the system for referral and counterreferral among the various levels functions adequately.

Grass-roots management has become the mechanism for community participation, which functions at the central level through the National Committee of Support for the Plan, at the regional level through the intersectoral commissions, and at the district level through health commissions. From an operational standpoint, community participation is accomplished through the activities of local health workers who, after receiving adequate training and support, provide crucial services in maternal and child health. In 1990, 1000 local health workers were trained, in addition to 100 lay midwives and 1000 women leaders.

In 1989, 37.9% of pregnant women, 28.8% of deliveries, and 28.8% of infants were attended by trained personnel. In 1990, 12.2% of the women of childbearing age were using contraceptive methods, and 60.3% of pregnant women received tetanus toxoid.

Immunization coverage of children under 1 year of age in 1990 was 48% for BCG, 41% for DPT, 50% for polio vaccine, and 53% for measles vaccine.

In 1988, 46% of the population was supplied with drinking water (77.36% in urban areas and 15.16% in rural areas), and 33.98% had adequate excreta disposal systems (55.44% in urban areas and 12.73% in rural areas).

Bolivia receives assistance for its activities from foreign national or multilateral organizations and carries out joint activities with its neighboring countries for the solution of various common problems.

BRAZIL

Demographic factors

In 1990, the population was estimated at 149 million, 26.2% of which lives in rural areas. Geographical distribution of the population is irregular, with a high concentration in the southern, southeastern, and midwestern regions. For 1985–1990, the annual rate of population growth was estimated at 1.9%; the birthrate at 26.7 per 1000; and fertility at 3.5 children per woman.

Socioeconomic factors

The illiteracy rate for the country is estimated at 22.2%. The per capita GDP in 1989 was estimated at US$2540, and the rate of inflation for 1980–1989 was an estimated 227.8% per year. According to 1984 data, 35% of the families in the country were living in poverty and 15% in extreme poverty. The unemployment rate for 1990 was estimated at 4.4%.

Health indicators

For 1985–1990, estimated total mortality was 7.8 per 1000; infant mortality, 63 per 1000 live births; and life expectancy at birth, 64.9 years.

The three leading causes of death are diseases of the circulatory system, external causes, and malignant neoplasms, with large variations from one geographical area to another. In 1989, 11.5% of all live born children had a birthweight of 2500 grams or less, 10.5% in urban areas and 14.8% in rural areas.

According to a survey carried out in 1989, 15.8% of children from 0 to 6 years of age showed low height-for-age.

Health care system

The constitution that came into effect in 1988 grants all Brazilians the right to health. The law also provides for the integration of public health services under a Unified Health Service. Among the actions taken to achieve this goal is the establishment of the National Health Foundation, which seeks to improve coordination, facilitate the planning process, and create the conditions for more efficient administrative management.

A process to decentralize health care services has been initiated through the transfer of federal services to the state and municipality levels.

Community participation is established by law at the level of the National Health Council and the state health councils, in which the communities are represented.

According to the Department of Statistics and Social Indicators, there were 32 450 health establishments in 1987, of which 24 174 (74.49%) were public. Of these, 6920 were hospitals (1149 public and 5771 private), with a total of 500 000 beds (107 694 public).

In 1988, the registry of professionals revealed that Brazil had 11.37 physicians, 6.55 dentists, 2.84 nurses, 1.55 nursing auxiliary technicians, 6.38 nursing auxiliaries, 2.59 pharmacists, 1.72 veterinarians, 0.81 nutritionists, and 4.8 psychologists per 10 000 population.

The distribution of resources varies widely in the country; they are highly concentrated in the most populated and developed areas; no national approach has been propounded for achieving more equitable distribution.

Total spending on health in 1989 represented 3.88% of the GDP, of which 2.48% corresponded to the public sector and 1.40% to the private.

Primary care

It is estimated that approximately 90% of the population has access to health care services for common diseases and traumas and that 65% of pregnant women are served by trained personal; however, no information is available with regard to delivery care. It is also estimated that approximately 40% of the population receives drugs free of charge every year.

In 1990, immunization coverage among children from 0 to 4 years of age was estimated at 78% for BCG, 81% for DPT, 93% for polio vaccine, and 78% for measles vaccine.

In 1988, it was estimated that 90.6% of the urban population had household water supply and 58.1% of the rural population had easy access to water. Of the urban population, 42.2% had sewerage connections and 89% had adequate excreta disposal services. Of the rural population, 29% had adequate excreta disposal.

Brazil has signed cooperation agreements with various countries, especially for the development of research and the training of personnel. These agreements have been made mainly with developed countries, (Belgium, Canada, Czechoslovakia, France, Germany, Italy, Japan, and the United States of America).

CANADA

Demographic factors

Canada's population for 1990 was estimated at 26 525 000, and the annual growth rate for 1985–1990 was estimated at 0.88%. Three-fourths of the population lives in urban communities. In 1990, 20.9% of the population was under 15 years of age, and 11.5% was 65 years of age or over. The birthrate recorded in 1987 was 14.4 per 1000, and the fertility rate for 1985–1990 was 1.7 children per woman.

Socioeconomic factors

For 1988–1989 the per capita GDP was US$19 020. Inflation for 1980–1989 was estimated at 4.6% per year. Urban unemployment in 1990 was 8.1%. In 1986, 83% of the population 15 years of age and over had completed more than nine years of schooling.

Health indicators

Total mortality registered in 1987 was 7.2 per 1000, and infant mortality in 1987 and 1988 was 7.2 per 1000 live births, with a postneonatal component of 2.6 per 1000 births. In 1988, maternal mortality was 0.5 per 10 000 live births.

Life expectancy at birth for 1985–1990 was 76.7 years.

Six percent of live born children had a birthweight of less than 2500 grams (5.5% for males and 6.5% for females).

The leading causes of death in 1988 were diseases of the circulatory system, malignant neoplasms, accidents and other violence, diseases of the respiratory system, and diseases of the digestive system.

Health care system

By constitutional mandate, the provision of personal health care services is the responsibility of the provinces and territories, except in the case of special groups, such as the indigenous populations and armed forces personnel, who come under federal jurisdiction.

The national health insurance plan guarantees medical and hospital care for all residents on a prepaid basis. Some provinces include certain additional benefits, such as dental care for children; optometric, dental, and psychological services; nontraditional medicine; home care; drugs; and preventive care.

A mechanism exists to provide for consultation and collaboration between the federal, provincial, and territorial governments in the area of health. Responsibility for financing the health services is also shared by these levels.

In the last decade, special emphasis has been placed on preventive care and health promotion activities.

During the First International Conference on Health Promotion, held in November 1986, Canada's Minister of Health and Welfare presented a strategy document that outlined the country's major targets for reducing health care inequalities and simultaneously increasing preventive care efforts and the ability to cope with chronic diseases and disability.

In 1988, there were 1244 hospitals in Canada with a total of 176 393 beds; of these facilities, 1096 hospitals and 170 366 beds belonged to the public sector.

In 1988, the country had 22.0 physicians, 80.8 nurses, 15.9 nursing assistants, 3.8 social workers, 5.3 dentists, 7.9 pharmacists, and 2.1 veterinarians per 10 000 population. It is believed that there is a surplus of physicians, and, consequently, many provinces have reduced enrollment in medical schools and graduate-level training programs.

Spending on health represented 8.9% of the GDP in 1989.

Primary care

The provincial, regional, and municipal authorities are responsible for primary care services, including the provision of drinking water and excreta disposal services, operation of public health programs, epidemiological surveillance of communicable diseases, health education, inspection of food-service establishments, home and hospital services for mothers and newborns, and management of school dental clinics.

Several strategies also have been developed for providing services to remote areas by such means as air ambulances and special health teams. The peripheral services are made up of referral networks coordinated at the provincial level.

Intersectoral cooperation in the area of health has increased notably in recent years, particularly with regard to campaigns against the use of tobacco; the strategy for control of drug abuse; the plan of action on health and the environment; the project for healthy communities; and the programs on family violence, the elderly, and AIDS. The project for healthy communities, aims at reducing inequalities in health care and raising awareness of environmental issues and health and safety in the workplace.

The contribution of volunteers is extremely important in Canada, especially regarding services to promote health and well-being. Nongovernmental organizations are invited to participate in the planning of health activities by providing information and proposing new orientations for the programs. Canada provides health assistance to developing countries and receives assistance from international institutions, especially for human resource training.

It is estimated that the entire population has access to the health services, and that all pregnant women and nursing infants, in addition to almost 100% of deliveries, are attended by trained personnel.

Seventy-five percent of children receive DPT and polio vaccines, and 85% are immunized against measles before the age of 2. The entire population has drinking water services, either supplied through household connection or at a distance of no more than 15 minutes on foot, and 85% has adequate excreta disposal systems.

CHILE

Demographic factors

The population for 1990 was estimated at 13 173 000, and the annual growth rate for 1985–1990 at 1.66%. Eighty-two percent of the country's inhabitants live in urban areas, and the capital city, Santiago, accounts for 39.7% of the country's total population. Thirty-one percent are under 15 years of age and 6% are 65 and older. The birthrate registered in 1989 was 23.4 per 1000 population, and the fertility rate was estimated at 2.7 children per woman.

Socioeconomic factors

The per capita GDP in 1990 was US$1890, and annual inflation for 1980–1989 was 20.5%. In 1990 unemployment was 6%. In 1987, 44% of the population was living below the poverty level, and 18% in extreme poverty.

Health indicators

In 1989, total reported mortality was 5.8 per 1000 population; child mortality for that year was 17.1 per 1000 live births, and was estimated at 18 per 1000 for 1985–1990. Maternal mortality was 4.1 per 10 000 live births.

Life expectancy at birth for 1985–1990 was 71.5 years.

The leading causes of mortality, in order of magnitude, are diseases of the heart, malignant neoplasms, external causes, diseases of the respiratory system, and diseases of the digestive system.

In 1989, 7.1% of newborns had a birthweight under 2500 grams, and 8.2% of surveyed children under 6 had a height-for-age deficit.

Health care system

The health sector is made up of the public and private subsectors, and the Ministry of Health leads the system. The National Health Services System of the public subsector is responsible for providing services to 80% of the population. The public sector's health activities are carried out by 26 functionally decentralized health services, each responsible for providing preventive and curative care to a given geographic area. These services also deal with occupational, school, and environ-mental health, and are effectively responsible for between 50% and 100% of the population, depending on the programs involved. There is, in addition, an environmental health service for the Metropolitan Region. The rest of the system provides predominantly curative care services.

In the 1980s, the Ministerial Regional Secretariats were established; they assumed the coordination of the public and private regional health services and advising the intendant of the region on health matters.

In 1990, a policy was adopted that aimed at developing and modernizing the health sector and meeting the most urgent needs of the population. Strategies to attain the goal of Health for All included improvements to the access to primary care, resolution of the hospital crisis, promotion of preventive care and health protection, improvements to the environment quality, and strengthening institutional capacity. The regulatory role of the Ministry of Health also was enhanced through the establishment of the Office of Supervision of the Provisional Health Institute. In 1990, the National Health Advisory Council also was established.

Chile has 40 900 hospital beds, 10 336 of which belong to the private sector. Human resources are distributed irregularly, and are heavily concentrated in the most developed areas. In 1990, the National System of Health Services had 6.4 physicians, 2 dentists, 0.2 pharmacists, 2.9 nurses, and 2.2 midwives per 10 000 population. The total number of physicians and nurses in the country per 10 000 population is estimated at 10.7 and 4.7, respectively; however, a large number of the nurses are unemployed.

Spending on health represented 2.5 of the GDP in 1990.

Primary care

Primary care services are basically provided by physicians' offices and rural health posts, which are largely administered by 241 of the 335 municipalities. The transfer of these services to the municipalities was an important step that began in 1980. The municipalities also are responsible for certain basic sanitation activities. The role of primary care is essentially one of health promotion and protection, and of sectoral articulation of the local community regarding health. In 1990, a program for strengthening primary care was launched.

In its first phase the program focuses on 62 urban physicians' offices in 22 communes, and it will be extended to 104 rural communes. In addition, measures have been taken to guarantee free access to primary care.

In order to increase coverage, 12 mobile units have been deployed to serve the population in the most underserved areas. Adult, oral, and mental health programs are also being expanded.

The most complex services support the most complex procedures through referral and counter-referral, and also carry out control and supervisory functions.

Primary Care Departments have been set up in both the Ministry of Health and in the health services, in order to ensure improved coordination.

Training activities have been carried out, including training for community leaders. Traditional community participation has mainly been expressed through charitable activities. More recently, inter-relationships with formal groups have been activated, and the training of community leaders and health monitors has been promoted.

In 1989, 99.8% of deliveries were attended in institutions, and 81.1% of young children were served by trained personnel. Immunization coverage in 1990 was 97% for BCG, 99% for DPT and polio vaccine, and 98% for measles vaccine.

In 1988, 85.97% of the total population had drinking water services (100% urban and 20.57% rural), and 83.44% had sanitary excreta disposal services (100% urban and 6.22 rural).

Some projects rely on bilateral and multilateral international cooperation.

COLOMBIA

Demographic factors

The estimated population in 1990 was 31 819 000, with an annual growth rate of 2.08% for 1985–1990. The population under 15 years of age accounts for 36.09% of the total, and those aged 65 and over represent 4.13%. Thirty-five percent of the population lives in rural areas. The estimated birthrate for 1985–1990 was 27.4 per 1000, and the fertility rate, 3.1 children per woman in 1990.

Socioeconomic factors

The per capita GDP in 1990 was US$1200. Inflation reached 24.3% for 1980–1989. Urban unemployment was 10.3% in 1990. In 1985, 13.3% of the total population was illiterate.

Health indicators

Total mortality for 1985–1990 was estimated at 6.1 per 1000, and infant mortality was 40.0 per 1000 live births; in 1989, infant mortality was reported to be 38 per 1000. Maternal mortality registered in 1989 was 4.0 per 10 000 live births. Life expectancy at birth is 68.2 years.

Mortality is seriously underreported, especially regarding children under 5 years of age.

In 1988, 12.8% of newborns weighed less than 2500 grams at birth.

During 1986–1989, it was reported that 13% of children under 5 years of age had weight-for-age deficits, and 4.9% had height-for-age deficits.

In 1989, the leading causes of death were malignant neoplasms, homicides, ischemic heart disease, other forms of heart disease, and cerebrovascular accidents. The leading reasons reported for consultation were other diseases of the genitourinary system, acute respiratory infections, diseases of the oral cavity, injuries, and intestinal infections.

Health care system

The health system is made up of the public, the private, and the social security subsectors, all of which compose the National Health System. The health sector is directed by the Ministry of Health. Only 16% of the population benefits from some kind of social security system.

In 1990, a law was enacted to restructure the National Health System.

Colombia's health policy emphasizes the following:

—Basic health care and environmental measures for families and the community, including extension of coverage, emphasis on preventive care, creation of a health-oriented culture, and organization and mobilization of community resources.
—The unification of the health system and the system of universal public health insurance.
—Decentralization and municipalization of health care management.
—Efficient and effective management of health care institutions.
—Rationalization of the production and distribution of drugs and health supplies as a means of ensuring quality and reducing costs.
—Improvement of the quality of municipal drinking water and sanitation services.
—Restructuring of profiles for the training of human resources.
—Improvement of disease control and epidemiological surveillance.

In recent years, attention has focused on the development of research, especially in areas that deal with the administration of health care and the procedures followed in providing primary care.

In 1989, the public sector had 661 hospitals with 29 427 beds, 784 health centers and 2492 health posts; the social security system had 27 hospitals with 2853 beds; and the private sector, 194 hospitals with 10 673 beds.

In 1989, the country had 9.2 physicians, 4.3 dentists, 2.7 nurses, 9.5 nursing auxiliaries, and 3.3 veterinarians per 10 000 population; however, distribution of the professional resources was largely concentrated in the most developed areas.

Primary care

In 1986, dialogue and consensus-building was initiated with community representatives, in order to identify health needs, formulate solutions, and carry out activities; however, the process has not yet been sufficiently generalized.

In 1988, a general primary care strategy was in effect, but in 1990, strategies were revised in conjunction with the restructuring of the National Health System and the move toward decentralization. Nongovernmental organizations traditionally have collaborated with the health sector in the development of certain health programs. In 1989, a decree by the Office of the President of the Republic established the legal standards for the establishment, composition, and operation of Community Participation Committees, which, among other functions, participate in drug control; preventive care programs; monitoring the referral and counterreferral system; and diagnosing, programming, monitoring and evaluating the health services.

Community health officials have conducted scanty actions, mainly because activities must be carried out largely outside the normal working hours for which they were hired and no adequate incentives have been provided for this kind of work, particularly regarding remuneration.

In 1989, 58.9% of pregnant women and an equal percentage of deliveries were attended by trained personal, and 27.1% of pregnant women were vaccinated with tetanus toxoid. In 1990, it was reported that 40% of the women of childbearing age were using some kind of contraceptive method, whereas according to 1988 information, 64.8% of women of childbearing age with live-in partners were using contraceptives.

Immunization coverage among infants aged 1 year or under in 1990 was 95% for BCG, 87% for DPT, 93% for polio vaccine, and 82% for measles vaccine.

In 1988, 87.5% of the total population had drinking water services (87.78% in urban areas and 86.81% in rural areas), and 65.06% had adequate excreta disposal systems (84.64% in urban areas and 17.58% in rural areas).

COSTA RICA

Demographic factors

The population of the country in 1990 was estimated at 3 015 000, and the annual growth in the same year was 2.64%. A total of 36.2% of the population is under 15 years of age, and 4.2% is 65 or over; 54.5% live in rural areas. The birthrate in 1989 was 25.5 per 1000; the fertility rate for 1985–1990 was estimated at 3.3 children per woman.

Socioeconomic factors

The per capita GDP in 1990 was US$1940. The annual inflation rate for 1980–1989 was 24.8%. In 1990, urban unemployment reached 5.4%. Illiteracy in 1990 was estimated at 7.4%.

Health indicators

In 1989, the total death rate was 3.8 per 1000 population, and infant mortality was 13.9 per 1000 live births, which represents a decline from the 17% per 1000 reported for 1985–1990. In 1989, mortality in children aged 1 to 4 years old was registered at 0.7 per 1000, and maternal mortality was 3.0 per 10 000 live births. Life expectancy at birth for 1985–1990 was estimated at 74.7 years. In 1987, 6.2% of newborns weighed under 2500 grams at birth, and 25.8% of children under 6 years of age showed weight-for-age deficits.

In 1989, the leading causes of death were acute myocardial infarction, other forms of ischemic heart disease, malignant neoplasms of the stomach, certain conditions arising in the perinatal period, and congenital anomalies.

Health care system

The National Health Law establishes that good health is in the public interest, and makes health a responsibility of the State, specifically the Executive Branch through the Ministry of Health. Health sector institutions function according to regionalization and sectoral division of responsibilities. The Ministry of Health is responsible for health promotion, disease prevention, and environmental protection; the Costa Rican Social Security Fund (CCSS) is charged with activities relating to the recovery of health, rehabilitation, and contributing to the Ministry's health promotion and preventive care activities; the National Insurance Institute is responsible for the care, rehabilitation, and compensation of all people covered under policies providing protection in the event of occupational injuries and motor vehicles accidents; and the Costa Rican Institute of Water Supply and Sewerage Systems is responsible for the drinking water supply and sewerage services. In December 1987, an agreement was signed between the Ministry and the CCSS for integrating the programming and use of their resources and coordinating their efforts and activities; in 1989, they began a joint process of annual operational planning at the local health systems level.

The institutional mechanism established for incorporating health targets into Costa Rica's socioeconomic development policies and programs is the National Planning Law, enacted in 1974. Intrasectoral coordination of the health sector is implemented by the National Health Council and the sector's Executive Secretariat. In recent years, there has been a strong political trend toward administrative regionalization, decentralization, and deconcentration. The National Planning Law created regions and decentralized planning and administration levels, assigning legal functions to them and providing for the participation of the various sectors.

The General Rules of the National Health System, established by Executive Decree in November 1989, expressly stipulate the functions and responsibilities of the sector's institutions. The fundamental policy of health for all advocates the State's political commitment as a whole, concerted effort by the social and economic sectors in order to achieve national and community development, equitable distribution of resources, participation by the community in shaping its future in health and socioeconomic terms, and technical and economic cooperation with other countries.

The national policies defined for 1990–1994 include seven major areas of action:

—Health promotion and disease control;
—Health care for special groups that assigns priority to marginalized population groups and indigenous communities, and concentrates actions in the areas that are most depressed and that have the worst health conditions in the country;
—Environmental health;

—Social promotion and participation;
—Development and strengthening of the health systems;
—Development of human resources; and
—Strengthening of physical and technological infrastructure.

The National Surveillance System has progressed in terms of epidemiological surveillance of reportable diseases, operational surveillance, and financial accounting.

In 1989, there were 1956 health establishments in Costa Rica, of which 1669 were operated by the Ministry of Health: 578 specialized in nutrition, 140 in dentistry, and 951 in comprehensive health care. Of the latter, 494 were health posts, 325 community health areas, 93 health centers, and 39 mobile medical care units. The Costa Rican Social Security Fund had 29 hospitals and 237 outpatient clinics. The National Insurance Institute had 16 medical clinics, a consultation center, and a rehabilitation center. In the same year, there were 2.4 hospital beds and 107 hospital discharges per 1000 population.

In 1991, there were 10.3 physicians, 3.6 dentists, 5 nurses, 22.7 nursing auxiliaries, 1.8 veterinarians, 0.06 sanitation engineers, and 2.2 local or village health workers per 10 000 population.

In 1989 public spending on health represented 5.8% of the GDP.

Primary care

Programs have been designed within the Ministry of Health that are clearly oriented toward primary care, such as programs on rural and community health, supplementary food and nutrition, monitoring of growth and development, child survival, early stimulation, dental care, and basic sanitation. The Costa Rican Social Security Fund has programs that focus on essential primary care for diseases that are highly prevalent in the epidemiological profile of the country.

In addition, an attempt is being made to coordinate the programs within the National Health System, incorporating the philosophy of primary care into integrated local health systems with special emphasis on local programming.

In order to redirect and reinforce the gains already made in primary care, activities have been carried out and continue to be carried out to strengthen programming at all levels, with special emphasis on the local level. These activities include building an effective local information system; strengthening community participation, communication, and collective education; formulating and implementing a sound legal framework for primary care; developing and strengthening local health systems; and developing comprehensive programming for the sector.

The Ministry of Health has always considered community participation to be fundamentally important. The National Program for Community Participation in Health aims at increasing community solidarity and encouraging community participation in health matters. This program envisions the realization of three types of communal efforts—analysis, planning, and evaluation and follow-up. Voluntary community participation has manifested itself in various ways, as exemplified by the activities of lay midwives (since 1954), health workers (since 1973), nutrition committees (since 1951), health committees (since 1973), the Cantonal Health Associations (since 1978), the Health and Social Security Boards (since 1983), and participation by community representatives in the Basic Technical Councils at the local level.

Costa Rica receives assistance from both governmental and nongovernmental institutions to carry out some of its health programs, and it also maintains cooperation ties with neighboring countries.

It is estimated that 100% of urban and concentrated rural populations and 95% of the scattered rural populations have access to health services. In 1989, 91% of pregnant women and 93.8% of deliveries were attended by trained personnel. In 1986, 91% of infants also received care from trained personnel. A total of 6.7% of pregnant women were vaccinated with tetanus toxoid in 1990. In children under 1 year of age the coverage rates were 92% for BCG, 95% for DPT, 95% for polio vaccine, and 90% for measles vaccine.

In 1988, 93.58% of the total population had drinking water services (100% of the urban population and 83.90% of the rural population); and 97.17% of the total population had adequate excreta disposal systems (100% of the urban population and 92.94% of the rural population).

CUBA

Demographic factors

In 1990, the estimated population was 10 324 000, and the annual growth rate for 1985–1990 was 0.75%. In 1989, 27.2% of the population resided in rural areas. A total of 23.1% of the population was under 15 years of age and 8.5% was 65 or older. The birthrate registered in 1989 was 17.6 per 1000, and the fertility rate for 1985–1990, 1.8 children per woman.

Socioeconomic factors

The per capita Gross Social Product at constant prices in 1989 was 2533 Cuban pesos. Unemployment for the same year was estimated at 6%. Of the working-age population, which constitutes 52.1% of the total, 70% is actively employed, 1.5% is seeking work for the first time, and the remainder is made up of students, housewives, and people engaged in domestic and other occupations.

Health indicators

In 1989, total mortality was 6.4 per 1000 population; infant mortality was 11.1 per 1000 live births (neonatal, 7.2 per 1000 and postneonatal, 3.9 per 1000). Maternal mortality was 2.92 per 10 000 live births and mortality in children aged 1–4 years was, 0.7 per 1000.

Life expectancy at birth for 1985–1990 was 75.2 years. In 1989, 7.3% of newborns weighed less than 2500 grams. The leading causes of death are diseases of the heart, malignant neoplasms, cerebrovascular diseases, accidents, and influenza and pneumonia. In infants under 1 year old, the five leading causes are certain causes originating in the perinatal period, congenital anomalies, influenza and pneumonia, enteritis and other diarrheal diseases, and accidents.

Health care system

Cuba's National Health System is unified, comprehensive, regionalized, and decentralized; it is administered and financed by the State. It comprises three administrative levels that reflect the country's political and administrative divisions: the Central Government, 14 provinces, and 169 municipalities. The Ministry of Public Health is the regulatory organism, and its role includes per-forming methodological, coordination, and control functions; it is directly responsible for the research institutes, the medical institutes and schools of medicine, some national hospitals, and the national production and distribution of drugs. The provincial and municipal health offices are administered by provincial and municipal peoples' assemblies (local governments), which give the health offices their financing, supplies, work force, and maintenance. In terms of methodology, they come under the Ministry of Public Health. The National Health System delivers health care services to the population through a network of facilities that can provide care of varying degrees of complexity. There are four levels of services: national, provincial, municipal, and health area.

The current development strategy aims at refining preventive health care and health promotion; developing the network of units and medical specialties; continuing to improve the system of training, specialization, and continuing education of human resources for public health; prioritizing and supporting scientific research; and developing the pharmaceutical industry and the manufacture of medical equipment.

The information required to conduct evaluations is obtained from the Statistics Information System, which is subdivided into a National Statistics Information Subsystem that includes economic and social information for the general administration of the country and a Complementary Statistics Information Subsystem that includes information more specifically related to the health sector. The national research policy is set by the Academy of Sciences for all the central organizations of the Cuban economy. The Ministry of Public Health then establishes lines of research to be carried out through a national plan that is primarily concerned with the health needs of the population and the development needs of the country as a whole.

Cuba has 208 urban hospitals, 104 of which are general hospitals; in addition, there are 66 rural hospitals, and a total of 59 667 beds; 392 urban and 28 rural polyclinics; 66 urban and 163 rural medical posts; 5161 urban and 1885 rural family physician's offices; and 161 urban and 2 rural oral health clinics. In 1990, there were 36.5 physicians and 47.4 health technicians per 10 000 population.

In 1989, 3.39% of the Gross Social Product was spent on health. Of total spending on health,

89.8% went to local services and 30.5% to primary care.

Primary care

Since 1984, a family physician system has been in effect. This system is community-based and, from the standpoint of administration and scientific and technical support, is part of the polyclinic and rural hospital systems. The family doctor, along with the polyclinics, constitutes the basic unit of primary; they provide the auxiliary services for diagnosis and consultation in the various medical specialties. In 1990, family doctors provided care for 56.7% of the population; the remainder was covered by the polyclinics and rural hospitals. A system is in place for referral and counterreferral of patients among the various levels of health care, and there is coordination among all government sectors at the national, provincial, and municipal levels.

The community participates fully in determining health needs, carrying out actions, and managing health care. Family doctors and nurses hold semiannual assemblies on health diagnosis with the population they serve.

Cuba gives to and receives cooperation in the area of health from several countries, and also receives support from international organizations.

The entire population has access to health services. In 1989, 100% of infants, pregnant women, and deliveries were served by trained personnel; 15.1 prenatal visits were provided for each delivery, and 99.8% of deliveries were handled in institutions. Ninety-five percent of pregnant women received tetanus toxoid. In 1987, according to a national fertility survey, 50.4% of fertile women with live-in partners were using effective contraceptive methods, while 27.7% were using ineffective methods. Immunization coverage of infants under 1 year of age in 1990 was 98% for BCG, 92% for DPT, 94% for polio vaccine, and 94% for measles vaccine.

In 1990, 100% of the population of Cuba had drinking water services, 66% through household connections; the remainder had drinking water at a distance of not more than 200 meters in urban areas and at less than one hour's distance in rural areas. Twenty-eight percent of the country's population has sewerage services (38% of the urban population and 3% of the rural), and the remainder of the urban and rural population has some other system for excreta disposal.

DOMINICAN REPUBLIC

Demographic factors

The population in 1990 was estimated at 7 170 000 of which 39.62% reside in rural areas. The growth rate for 1985–1990 was estimated at 2.22%. Persons under 15 years of age constituted 38.6% of the population in 1988. The birthrate was estimated at 31.3 per 1000 population per year for 1985–1990 and the fertility rate, at 3.8 children per woman.

Socioeconomic factors

The per capita GDP was US$790 in 1989, and inflation during 1980–1989 was 19.1% per year. An estimated 20% of the total population is illiterate, and the rate of urban unemployment in 1990 was estimated at 29%.

Health indicators

Total mortality for 1985–1990 was estimated at 6.8 per 1000 population per year, and infant mortality, at 65 per 1000 live births. Maternal mortality in 1990 was recorded at 9.0 per 10 000 live births. Life expectancy at birth for 1985–1990 was 65.9 years.

The leading causes of mortality are diseases of the heart, certain conditions originating in the perinatal period, malignant neoplasms, cerebrovascular disease, accidents, and influenza and pneumonia.

The disease most frequently reported is diarrhea; this situation, together with the high recorded frequency of dysentery, parasitic diseases, typhoid fever, and hepatitis, makes orally transmitted diseases a significant problem.

In 1989, birthweights for 13.7% of the live births were under 2500 grams.

Among users of the Ministry of Public Health and Social Welfare health services in 1990, malnutrition was found in 4.17% of children under 5 years of age, in 7.32% of the children under 1 year of age, and in 3.30% of the children aged 1–4 years.

Health care system

The system is divided between the public and private sectors. The public sector health system consists of the Ministry of Public Health and Social Welfare (SESPAS), the Dominican Social Security Institute (IDSS), the Social Security Institute of the Armed Forces and the National Police (INSFAPOL), and the National Council for Population and Family. The private sector comprises several nonprofit institutions, which cover a high percentage of the tertiary care in many medical specialties, and the for-profit sector, which offers predominantly curative services.

The Ministry is the regulatory agency for health actions; it consists of a central level that has political, technical, and normative roles; a regional level (comprising eight regions) with managerial, supervisory, and control duties; and an area level that is basically operational.

The current strategy for health, established in 1990, is oriented toward deconcentration and decentralization, mobilization of national resources, selective concentration of resources, formulation of projects, reduction of the bureaucracy, financing and the search for alternative sources of financing, and community participation.

The Ministry has initiated actions aimed at achieving coordination with IDSS and other institutions to strengthen infrastructure, especially of local services. To that end, a technical administrative unit responsible for developing mechanisms for intersectoral coordination was created within Ministry, and policies and strategies were formulated to achieve this objective.

Services are delivered in a hierarchical system, with a first level consisting of clinics and health workers and supervisors, a second level made up of the health subcenters and the local and area hospitals, and a third level that includes the regional and national hospitals.

In 1990, the Ministry had 8 specialized hospitals, 7 regional hospitals, 26 area hospitals, 78 health subcenters, 506 rural clinics, and 63 dispensaries and medical offices. It also had 5654 health workers and 847 supervisors.

In 1988, the country had 5.7 physicians and 15.4 nurses per 10 000 population. Health professionals are concentrated at the levels of greater complexity, but efforts are being made to increase their numbers in the local services.

Primary care

The overall policy for 1991–1995 focuses on preventive actions, maintenance of the health infrastructure, control of epidemic diseases, reorganization of the sector, use of appropriate technology, and community participation.

A health education program on AIDS that deals with the Expanded Program on Immunization is being developed for the population. The biologicals for the Immunization Program are offered continuously and free-of-charge in all health establishments.

The population served by the Ministry (more than 60% of the total) is provided free services, and the necessary drugs are donated to low-income patients. In addition, drugs are available at low cost in the local drug stores that are found throughout the country.

Community participation results in the work of almost 6000 health workers and the establishment of many Health Improvement Committees.

In 1990, 43.35% of pregnant women and 44% of deliveries were attended by trained personnel.

In 1990, immunization coverage among children under 1 year of age reached 68% for BCG, 96% for DPT, 90% for polio vaccine, and 96% for measles vaccine.

In 1988, 51.51% of the total population (67.68% in urban areas and 28.43% in rural) had drinking water and 59.74% had adequate excreta disposal systems (76.55% in urban areas and 35.75% in rural).

The Dominican Republic receives assistance from other countries and from international organizations to carry out some activities; it also engages in joint actions with Haiti to address certain health problems common to both countries.

ECUADOR

Demographic factors

The population for 1990 was estimated at 10 547 000, and the growth rate for 1985–1990 was 2.50% per year. Of the total population, 43.09% of the population lives in rural areas and 40% is under 15 years of age. The birthrate for 1985–1990 was estimated at 32.3 per 1000 population, and the fertility rate was 4.1 children per woman.

Socioeconomic factors

The per capita GDP in 1990 was US$1010, and inflation for 1980–1989 was 34.4% per year. In 1990, 14.6% of the population was illiterate, and in 1989, urban unemployment was estimated at 7.9%.

Health indicators

Officially reported total mortality in 1987 was 5.2 per 1000 population; however, a special survey estimated this figure at 7.6 for the same year. Infant mortality was estimated at 63 per 1000 births per year for 1985–1990. The official reported rate was 44.7 in 1988 and 48 in 1987; however, for the latter year, according to the same special survey, it was approximately 60 per 1000. Mortality for children aged 1–4 was 3.44 per 1000 in 1988. Life expectancy at birth for 1985–1990 was estimated at 65.4 years. Maternal mortality in 1988 was reported to be 15.6 per 10 000 live births.

The leading causes of death registered in 1987 were intestinal infectious diseases; pneumonia; cerebrovascular diseases; bronchitis, emphysema, and asthma; traffic accidents; ischemic heart disease; tuberculosis; malignant neoplasms of the stomach; and homicides. Regarding morbidity, it should be mentioned that malaria remains a persistent problem.

Health care system

The public subsystem is made up of the Ministry of Public Health, the Ecuadorian Social Security Institute (IESS), the Armed Forces Health Service, the Welfare Board of Guayaquil, the National Institute for Children and Families, and the Ministry of Social Welfare; the first two are the most important entities in terms of installed capacity, infrastructure, and coverage. The private sector is made up of nonprofit institutions and several for-profit hospitals, clinics, and physicians' offices.

The health policy is framed around five fundamental lines of action within the 1989–1992 National Health Plan: comprehensive family and community health, food and nutrition, basic sanitation, supply of drugs, and improvement of hospital care. The Plan underscores the importance of implementation of the National Health System, coordination between training institutions and employers of human resources, integration of all the sectoral institutions, and community participation. In addition, it emphasizes a reorientation of the actions and programs for outpatient care and comprehensive prioritized care for high-risk population groups. The activities of the National Health Council, an advisory body that was established in order to group the sector's institutions have helped to strengthen coordination.

Until 1988, the sector was, for all practical purposes, centralized; since then, however, studies have been carried out to establish priority areas for decentralization and to propose the most viable mechanisms for achieving it. To this end, manuals were prepared outlining procedures for the decentralized management of finances, human resources, and the supply of material resources. In terms of surveillance and evaluation of the health system, obstacles that essentially derive from the need for an integrated information system, the lack of definition of certain indicators, and the isolated development of evaluation subsystems have been identified.

In 1987, Ecuador had 2260 health establishments: 380 were hospitals and 1880 were outpatient facilities, including 66 urban health centers, 289 health posts, 789 rural health subcenters, and 736 urban and rural clinics. A total of 16 426 beds were available, 65% of which belonged to the public sector. In 1990, the number of establishments increased to 2743, of which 2349 were outpatient facilities.

In 1988, Ecuador had 10.5 physicians, 1.3 dentists, 3 nurses, 12.2 nursing auxiliaries, 0.3 social workers, and 0.4 midwives per 10 000 population.

Primary care

In the Ministry of Public Health, the concept of primary care has been disseminated and applied at the first level of care and the first three levels of complexity (health posts, subcenters, and health centers) through health promotion and protection activities. Although the entire population has not yet been covered in an equitable manner, the launching of the Comprehensive Family and Community Health Program over the last two years has introduced health services into the marginal urban neighborhoods in the principal cities. Coverage is now being expanded toward critical rural areas.

IESS, through the Rural Social Security System, covers 50% of the rural population, and has developed programs for health promotion, preventive care, and basic rural sanitation. In order to cover the other 50% of this population, compulsory insurance was instituted for agricultural workers.

Although no two-way referral system has been implemented, continuous support is being provided for outpatient establishments by the establishments of greater complexity.

Community participation has become more obvious in the rural areas, especially in terms of environmental sanitation and construction of health institutions.

In 1988, 47.4% of pregnant women, 25.8% of deliveries, 65.1% of children under 1 year of age, and 8.9% of children aged 1–4 received care from trained personnel. Among women of childbearing age (which includes pregnant women), 2% had received tetanus toxoid and 31.7% were using contraceptive methods.

In 1990, immunization coverage of infants under 1 year of age was 88% for BCG, 68% for DPT, 67% for polio vaccine, and 61% for measles vaccine.

In 1988, 57% of the population had drinking water services (75.11% in urban areas and 36.97% in rural areas) and 56.43% had adequate excreta disposal systems (75.24% in urban areas and 34.19% in rural areas).

Ecuador receives cooperation from other countries and multilateral agencies for the execution of some of its health programs.

EL SALVADOR

Demographic factors

The population was estimated at 5 252 000 in 1990; 44% is urban and 45% is under 15 years of age. For 1985–1990 the growth rate was estimated at 1.75%, the birthrate at 34.6 per 1000 population, and the fertility rate at 4.5 children per woman.

Socioeconomic factors

The per capita GDP was US$1070 in 1990 and the annual rate of inflation for 1980–1989 was 16.8%. In 1970, the illiteracy rate for those over 15 years of age was 42%; by 1990 it was estimated that it had declined to 27%.

Health indicators

For 1985–1990 total mortality was estimated at 8.64 per 1000 and infant mortality at 59 per 1000 live births. In 1989, maternal mortality was 12.7 per 10 000 live births. Life expectancy at birth was estimated at 62.2 years for 1985–1990.

In 1987, the leading causes of death were certain conditions arising in the perinatal period, homicides, intestinal infections, cerebrovascular diseases, and pneumonia. The leading reasons for consultation were normal pregnancy, ill-defined intestinal infections, the common cold, intestinal parasitism, and acute upper respiratory infections.

In 1990, 15.03% of those born in hospitals and 8.05% of those born with a midwife in attendance weighed less than 2500 grams.

An evaluation of the food and nutrition situation carried out in 1988 revealed height-for-age deficits in 11.9% of children aged 0–11 months, 28.6% of those aged 12–17 months, 37.5% of those aged 18–23 months, 42.3% of those aged 2 years, 30.9% of those aged 3 years, 34.1% of those aged 4 years, and 29.9% of those aged 5 years.

Health care system

There are 70 health-related institutions in the country. In the government sector, the Ministry of Public Health and Social Welfare, where the Constitution has charged with safeguarding the health of the entire population, serves 85% of the population. The other government agency, the Salvadoran Social Security Institute, serves the population affiliated with it. In 1989 and in 1990, the budget of the Ministry constituted 0.94% of the GDP; 11.44% and 13.30%, respectively, were allotted to local services.

A Socioeconomic Development Plan has been prepared, covering the education, health and nutrition, housing, comprehensive family care, social welfare, and labor sectors. In the health and nutrition sector the specific policies are:

—Channeling of health spending to improve care and expand the coverage of the primary health services and to increase coverage in the area of comprehensive maternal and child health.

—Modernizing the public health services administration to increase the effectiveness and the administrative and operating efficiency of the Ministry in order to improve the services and the use of available resources, and structuring the National Health System.

—Channeling food aid toward vulnerable groups living in extreme poverty.

—Modernizing food aid administration, improving the planning and coordinating mechanisms, and making the group feeding programs functional.

There are no reliable data available on human resources in health, which is known to be unevenly distributed, with high concentrations in the capital, especially physicians.

The National Health Plan for 1991 to 1994 includes the following strategies: extension of coverage to the entire population, enhancement of the capability of the various levels of care, decentralization, institutional development, financial strengthening, interinstitutional and intersectoral coordination, and coordination of international cooperation.

Primary care

The concept of primary care, although it has been accepted as a goal, is understood in different ways, even within the same levels (central, regional, and local). The health care services function in an isolated fashion, and the population is not totally covered. Moreover, patient referral to the other levels is not well structured.

The promotion of community participation has involved such efforts as the establishment of open councils that can identify needs, the partial delegation of responsibility for the execution and maintenance of water and sanitation projects to the communities, the creation of mothers' clubs, the training of community health workers and leaders. However, no mechanisms are in place for the community to participate in planning.

Installed capacity has been improved, and efforts are being made to redistribute the resources at the national level in order to achieve better equity. The collaboration and training of lay midwives also is being sought as a way to improve care during delivery. In addition, programs in nutrition and oral health are being developed.

Health services are accessible to 95% of the population, and basic drugs are available to 70% of the population served by the Ministry. It is estimated that 35% of the children under 1 year of age receive care from trained personnel and that 34% of births are handled in institutions.

In 1990, immunization coverage among children under 1 year of age was 60% for BCG, 76% for DPT and polio vaccine, and 75% for measles vaccine; 40% of pregnant women received two or more doses of tetanus toxoid.

In 1989, 46% of the population was being supplied with drinking water, 94% in urban areas and 10% in rural areas. Sewerage systems covered 68% of the urban population, while 33% of the rural population had latrines.

GUATEMALA

Demographic factors

The population in 1990 was estimated at 9 197 000. For 1985–1990 the annual rate of population growth was estimated at 2.88%. In 1987, 67.3% of the population lived in rural areas and 46% was under 15 years of age.

According to the 1981 census, 41.9% of the population is indigenous, with unequal distribution in the different departments. The birthrate reported for 1987 was 36.5 per 1000 population, and total fertility for 1985–1990 was estimated at 5.8 children per woman.

Socioeconomic factors

The per capita GDP for 1990 was US$910 and the annual rate of inflation for 1980–1989 was 13.4%. The urban unemployment rate was 6.4% in 1990.

Health indicators

Total mortality reported for 1987 was 8.1 per 1000 population. Infant mortality for 1985–1990 was estimated at 59 per 1000 live births per year; the figure recorded for 1988 was 51.3.

Life expectancy at birth for 1985–1990 was 62.0 years.

The leading causes of death are diarrheal diseases, acute respiratory infections, malnutrition, acute myocardial infarction, and accidents. The leading causes of morbidity recorded for 1986 by the Ministry of Public Health and Social Welfare's services were acute respiratory infections, intestinal parasitic infections, diarrheal syndrome, nutritional deficiency, and diseases of the skin. In the Guatemalan Social Security Institute (IGSS), the most frequent reasons for consultation were diseases of the respiratory system, infectious and parasitic diseases, and diseases of the digestive system.

Health care system

The health system comprises the Ministry of Public Health and Social Welfare, the Guatemalan Social Security Institute, the municipalities, the Military Health Department, the University of San Carlos, and the private sector.

The health policies for 1989 and 1990 included: increased coverage; environmental protection, conservation, and improvement; food and nutrition; institutional development and administration of the sector; and development of the physical infrastructure of the health sector. During this period, the National Commission on Oral Health was created; an effort was made to maintain an adequate supply of generic drugs in the health centers and posts; efforts were intensified to increase immunization coverage; and agreements were signed with international and national organizations in the area of health.

In 1989, Regional Health Administrations were created, which made it possible to group authorities from health areas and districts, as well as public and private institutions of the sector. However, it has not been possible to achieve their consolidation, although advances have been made in budgetary deconcentration.

The information system is fragmented and suffers from overall delays in reporting. In addition, there is no office responsible for systematic evaluation.

The Ministry of Public Health and Social Welfare spent 1.11% of the GDP in 1990 and utilized 8.46% of its budget for local services.

In 1989, the country had 67 hospitals with 7511 beds and in 1988 it had 1.46 physicians, 0.16 dentists, 1.27 nurses, 6.35 nursing auxiliaries, 0.39 sanitation inspectors, 0.67 laboratory workers, and 0.62 rural health technicians per 10 000 population.

Primary care

There have been efforts to achieve the integration of the different sectors involved: personnel from the various levels of the national health system, the national planning system, the community, the private sector, and the nongovernmental organizations. Ministry personnel from the first and second levels of care are carrying out actions that permit direct contact between the community and the health services. The IGSS is carrying out a program of primary care in one of the country's departments.

Regional Councils of Urban and Rural Development have been established, with representation from the Ministry; the municipalities, the cooperatives, and nongovernmental organizations from each region; and the national planning body. Their objective is to coordinate efforts of the public and private sectors to facilitate the development of the different regions. The National Health Council and, at the local level, the Health Management Committees also have been created, and efforts are under way to make them operational.

Community participation is carried out with groups and individuals through collaborators such as rural health workers, traditional midwives, and volunteers. However, the community does not participate in the programming and evaluation of health activities.

Despite efforts to promote primary care, hospitals remain as the establishments that have the greatest demand for human resources, and, thus, they are the best staffed health care facilities.

Trained personnel serve 33.98% of pregnant women and attend 22.58% of deliveries; 26% of the women of childbearing age use some method of contraception; and 12% of pregnant women receive tetanus toxoid.

Immunization coverage among children under 1 year of age in 1990 was 62% for BCG, 66% for DPT, 74% for polio vaccine, and 68% for measles vaccine.

Investment in sanitation works has increased, especially in the construction of rural water supply systems. In 1988, 60.17% of the population had drinking water (urban, 91.30%; rural, 41.19%) and 59.63% had adequate systems for excreta disposal (urban, 71.74%; rural, 47.91%).

The country receives international assistance for health activities, both from other countries and from multilateral organizations.

GUYANA

Demographic factors

The population in 1990 was estimated at 1 040 000, and the growth rate during 1985—1990 was 1.74% per year. Of the total population, 65.4% resides in rural areas; 42% is under 15 years of age; and 6% is over 65 years of age. The birthrate in 1986 was 23.8 per 1000 population and the fertility rate in 1985–1990 was estimated at 2.8 children per woman.

Socioeconomic factors

In 1990, the per capita GDP was US $340. The illiteracy rate is estimated at 3.6%.

Health indicators

Total mortality in 1986 was 7.9 per 1000 population. Infant mortality was 49.0 per 1000 live births, and in 1986, mortality among children aged 1–4 years was old 4.4 per 1000.

Life expectancy at birth for 1985–1990 was estimated at 69.7 years.

In 1986, it was reported that 12.0% of all live-born children had a birthweight of under 2500 grams; in 1984, the figure had been 19.5%.

A 1987 nutritional survey revealed that 23% of the children under 5 years of age showed signs of malnutrition. In 1986, it was reported that of those examined in this age group, 10.4% showed grade II or III of malnutrition according to the Gómez classification.

The leading causes of deaths registered in 1984 were cerebrovascular disease; diseases of the digestive system; diseases of the pulmonary circulation and other forms of heart disease, including ischemic heart disease; and diseases of the respiratory system.

Health care system

The health system consists mainly of public sector institutions, although private hospitals and physicians play an important role. Each region has a regional democratic council. The Ministry of Health carries out coordinating and normative functions and, in addition, provides direct preventive and health restoration services. The health services are regionalized, with the central level playing development, guidance, evaluation, and coordination roles. Efforts have been initiated to establish a regional information system that will include an information system for financial management.

The health system is organized into five levels: Level I is the community, where health activities are carried out by community health workers; Level II is the health center, which mainly utilizes health visitors and environmental health officials; Level III is the district, of which the district medical officer is the central authority; Level IV is the region, where care is provided in the principal specialties; and Level V is the National Referral Hospital in the capital.

The health policy mainly emphasizes the achievement of entire population's access to the best quality health care in order to facilitate the development of the entire country with more rapid progress in the least developed parts. Particular stress is laid on issues relating to women, children, and the elderly, as well as to agricultural development, designed to achieve self-sufficiency in food production, and to education in nutrition.

The health information system is deficient, primarily due to the lack of trained personnel.

Guyana has 65 health posts at Level I, 104 health centers, 8 district hospitals, 4 regional hospitals, 1 national referral hospital, and 3 specialized hospitals; the country also has 7 private hospitals.

In 1987, there were 2.0 physicians, 0.2 dentists, 9.8 nurses, 10.9 nursing auxiliaries, and 5.1 midwives per 10 000 population.

Spending on health represented 4.8% of the GDP in 1987. New ways of financing the health services are being sought.

Primary care

Efforts have been made to train health personnel in primary care.

There is a very good patient referral system among the different levels of health care. At the national level, the coordination of development plans is carried out through the Planning Commission, which includes a health sector official. At the regional level, there is a regional health management group, which comprises representatives from the community and all the relevant sectors of the administration.

It has been proposed that health committees be established in each community with fewer than

1000 inhabitants, and that in larger communities two or more committees, subdivided by area, be created. These committees would be responsible for the selection of individuals to be trained as community health workers and it is hoped that they would become involved in the planning and evaluation of the health services.

Some communities have participated in the construction of health services facilities, contributing labor or financing.

The participation of nongovernmental organizations has been oriented especially toward clinical activities.

The country receives international assistance for some of its health programs and carries out activities involving cooperation with neighboring countries.

It is estimated that 96% of the population has access to health services and that 95% of pregnant women, 93% of deliveries, and 98% of infants are attended by trained personnel. In 1987, it was reported that 47.5% of pregnant women received tetanus toxoid.

Immunization coverage for children under 1 year of age in 1990 was 85% for BCG, 83% for DPT, 79% for polio vaccine, and 73% for measles vaccine.

In 1988, 80.56% of the population (93.50% of the urban population and 74.31% of the rural) was being supplied with drinking water; the figures for excreta disposal systems were 85.58% for the total population, 84.55% for the urban population, and 86.08% for the rural population.

HAITI

Demographic factors

It was estimated that in 1990 the country had 6.5 million inhabitants, 70% of whom resided in rural areas. A high proportion of the population is young: 15% of the total are children under 5 years of age and 40% are under 15 years old. For 1985–1990, the annual growth rate was estimated at 2.3%, the birthrate at 36 per 1000 population per year, and the total fertility rate at 5 children per woman.

Socioeconomic factors

In 1989, the per capita GDP was estimated at US$360 and the inflation rate for 1980–1989 was 6.8%. The illiteracy rate is 47%. The rate of unemployment in 1990 was estimated at between 25% and 50%.

Health indicators

For 1985–1990, total mortality was estimated at 13 per 1000 population, infant mortality at 97 per 1000 live births per year, and maternal mortality at 23 per 10 000 live births.

Life expectancy at birth for 1985–1990 was estimated at 54.7 years.

The leading cause of consultation is diarrhea, which is also the leading cause of mortality. Other infectious and parasitic diseases such as malaria, intestinal parasitic diseases, pneumonia, tuberculosis, and typhoid fever are among the principal reasons for consultation. Malnutrition, AIDS, malaria, and pneumonia are also significant causes of mortality.

Among Haitian children, 10% have a birthweight of 2500 grams or less. It is reported that only 42% of the children have adequate weights for their ages according to the standard used.

Health care system

The health system includes the public, private nonprofit, and private for-profit sectors. The public sector is made up of the Ministry of Public Health and the Ministry of Population.

In 1990, the country's health services network had 477 establishments: 41 hospitals, 56 health centers with beds and 96 without beds, and 284 clinics. All of the urban population has easy access to services; however, only 35% of the rural population does, owing in large part to the geographical characteristics of some areas and to the scarcity of services. Financial accessibility is estimated at 30% to 35% for the urban area and 10% for the rural.

In 1989, the country had 1.64 physicians, 0.17 dentists, 1.24 nurses, 2.87 nursing auxiliaries, 0.35 laboratory technicians, and 0.70 health agents per 10 000 population. These resources are distributed unevenly, with high concentrations in the western region and the metropolitan area.

In March 1989, the Coordinating Unit for Priority Health Programs was created and, subsequently, the National Health Statistics Service was established. The first is responsible for the management of seven priority programs; the second is devoted to improving the information system, facilitating record keeping, and training personnel.

The priority programs are:

—Combating diarrheal dehydration and promoting breast-feeding.
—Immunizing against diseases preventable by vaccination.
—Stimulating maternal health and family planning.
—Combating malnutrition and nutritional diseases.
—Combating the most important endemic diseases.
—Combating tuberculosis.
—Fighting AIDS.

Executive decentralization and normative centralization have begun to be carried out, but there have been difficulties because of a lack of trained personnel at the peripheral levels, the scarcity of financial and material resources, political instability, and the inefficiency of the mechanisms for inter- and intrasectoral coordination.

The national plan of action that has been prepared sets objectives for each program (by department and by district), standards for activities, activity lists and schedules, and criteria for efficiency and effectiveness.

Primary care

The primary care strategy is being applied at all levels; however, it has not been possible to develop it fully, particularly because of problems relating to the personnel responsible. Community participation takes different forms—community leaders disseminate educational messages and participate in the selection of voluntary health agents and collaborators and the community also shares in other activities, such as the construction of clinics. As a way to increase participation, the Bureau of Health Education has been created, along with a subunit within the Coordinating Unit for Priority Programs, that is responsible for the preparation of a workable strategy for community involvement. Also, efforts are under way to train health agents and establish health committees and mothers' clubs.

The Planning and Evaluation Unit has been restructured in order to make planning more rigorous and increase the capacity for evaluation. In addition, the Ministry of Health has created committees for the prevention of diarrheal diseases and AIDS, an important effort designed to address these serious problems in the country.

Annual spending on health is estimated at US$23 per inhabitant; 20% is utilized for local health services.

In 1988, 41.80% of the population had drinking water services (55.47% in urban areas and 36.37% in rural) and 22.08% had adequate systems for excreta disposal (41.11% in urban areas and 14.52% in rural).

Immunization coverage among children under 1 year of age in 1990 was 72% for BCG, 41% for DPT, 40% for polio vaccine, and 31% for measles vaccine.

In 1988, 43% of pregnant women received prenatal care. Deliveries are attended at the institutional level in 20% of the cases, and the rest are generally attended by midwives.

Haiti receives support for its health programs from many developed and developing countries, as well as from multilateral organizations. It also has joint programs with its neighbor, the Dominican Republic.

HONDURAS

Demographic factors

The estimated population for 1990 was 5 138 000, and the growth rate for 1985–1990, at 3.18%. Of the total population, 56% lives in rural areas. According to the 1983 census, 45.9% of the population was under 15 years of age. The birthrate in 1987 was 38 per 1000 population and the total fertility rate for 1985–1990 was 5.6 children per woman.

Socioeconomic factors

In 1989, the per capita GDP was US$900 and the inflation rate for 1980–1989 was 4.7% per year. In 1988, 32% of the population was illiterate. The urban unemployment rate in 1990 was 7.1%. According to a survey carried out in 1988, 54.1% of the households had a monthly income that was not sufficient to meet basic food requirements.

Health indicators

Estimated total mortality for 1987 was 8.0 per 1000 population. Infant mortality for 1985–1990 was estimated at 68 per 1000 live births and in 1988 was recorded at 56 per 1000. In 1990, maternal mortality was 22.1 per 1000 live births.

Life expectancy at birth for 1985–1990 was estimated at 64.0 years.

In terms of morbidity, acute respiratory infections and intestinal infectious diseases are the leading reported causes. Malaria also continues to be a significant cause of morbidity in the country.

Of the children born in hospitals in 1988, 8.7% had a birthweight of under 2500 grams.

The National Nutrition Survey of 1987 revealed that 38% of children under 5 years old showed weight-for-age deficits and 3.9% and 44.7% had weight-for-height and height-for-age deficits, respectively.

Health care system

Both the public and private sectors provided health services. The public sector comprises the Ministry of Public Health and Social Welfare as the regulatory agency, the Honduran Social Security Institute (IHSS), the National Autonomous Water Supply and Sewerage Systems Service, the National Board of Social Welfare, and the Depart-ment of Medicine, Hygiene, and Occupational Safety in the Ministry of Labor. The network of services under the Ministry of Public Health is organized into eight health regions, which are subdivided into 35 health areas; these do not coincide with the country's territorial division.

The Ministry's plan of action encompasses the following areas of activity:

—Maximization of the effectiveness and efficiency of the health services, including administrative development, review and monitoring of the accessibility for marginalized groups, coordination with the IHSS, and development of referral institutions to support the local level.
—Maximization of the coverage, efficiency, and effectiveness of immunization programs.
—Identification, evaluation, and implementation of the drug program.
—Design of specific programs such as the improvement of the environment, nutrition, and feeding of specific segments of the population; systems of differential rates and monetary and in-kind subsidies; and community actions, among others.
—Design and administration of a system for monitoring the living conditions of deprived human groups.

Since 1988, efforts to improve the information network have intensified.

In 1989, the Ministry of Health's allotment represented 2.89% of the GDP; 40.6% of the budget is channeled into basic care.

In 1990, the country had 24 public and 15 private hospitals, 3 primary health care centers (with beds), 175 rural health centers with physicians, and 521 rural health centers without physicians. There was a total of 4000 beds.

Regarding human resources, the permanent registry of Ministry of Health personnel is being completed. During 1984–1988, there were 4.2 physicians, 1.6 nurses, and 0.8 dentists per 10 000 population. In 1990, the Ministry of Health and IHSS employed 9.65 nursing auxiliaries and 1.30 persons working in environmental sanitation per 10 000 population.

Primary care

Progress is being made in the development of local health systems. Community participation has been strengthened through the identification of strategies for each region designed to implement the policy of social participation, utilization of participatory action-oriented research, and the strengthening of voluntarism in health. Community drug funds have been established, and alternative sources of financing, such as direct payment for services received and the financing of services by private companies, are being sought.

It is estimated that 64% of the population has easy access to health services. In 1989, 77.7% of pregnant women, 63.3% of deliveries, and almost all infants received care from trained personnel; 20% of pregnant women received tetanus toxoid;

and 1.6% of the women of childbearing age used some contraceptive method.

In 1990, immunization coverage among children under 1 year of age was 71% for BCG, 84% for DPT, 87% for polio, and 90% for measles.

In 1988, 72.37% of the population had drinking water (89.37% in urban areas and 60.01% in rural) and 62.42% had adequate excreta disposal services (88.19% urban and 43.69% rural).

Honduras receives assistance from multilateral organizations and from several countries to carry out some health activities. In addition, it participates with neighboring countries in programs that address problems in the subregion.

JAMAICA

Demographic factors

In 1990, the population was estimated at 2 521 000 and the annual growth rate for 1985–1990, at 1.52%. In 1987, 52.2% of the population resided in rural areas and 38.3% was under 15 years of age. The birthrate for 1987 was 22.2 per 1000 population and the fertility rate for 1985–1990 was estimated at 2.9 children per woman.

Socioeconomic factors

The per capita GDP in 1989 was US$1260, and the inflation rate for 1980–1989 was estimated at 18.5% per year. For 1990, the rate of illiteracy was estimated at 18% and urban unemployment, at 18.2%.

Health indicators

In 1987, total mortality was 5.3 per 1000 population. For 1985–1990 infant mortality was estimated at 18 per 1000 live births per year and life expectancy at birth was 74.0 years.

Of the children born in public hospitals in 1988, 11.6% weighed less than 2500 grams.

A survey carried out in 1985 revealed that 6.6% of the children aged 59 months or less showed grade II malnutrition according to the Gómez classification; 0.3% showed grade III malnutrition.

In 1982, the leading causes of death recorded were cerebrovascular disease, diseases of the heart, malignant neoplasms, hypertension, and diabetes mellitus, followed by intestinal infectious diseases, and pneumonia and influenza.

Health care system

The Ministry of Health is the main supplier of health care services in the country, including those related to prevention, cure, environmental health, and the training in several health professions. The private sector also participates, but mostly in curative care. The public services are divided into four administrative levels: national, regional, county, and district.

The Government is committed to attaining the goal of health for all, and the application of primary health care is the basic strategy in that effort. To this end it seeks to:

—Ensure that the population of Jamaica has access to the health services and that compre-

hensive, efficient, acceptable care, provided in cooperation with the private sector, is offered to the entire population.

—Ensure services of high quality, through the establishment of quality control mechanisms for both public and private services.

—Rationalize the use of the health resources and design strategies to increase the budgetary sources for service delivery.

—Develop systems to recruit, train, and keep professionals in the health services.

—Consolidate, replace, or improve existing physical resources.

—Draft laws to protect public health.

—Ensure the availability of good-quality food in sufficient quantity to meet the nutritional needs of the population.

—Ensure preventive and curative care for vulnerable groups.

Efforts have been undertaken to cope with health services delivery problems, including political decisions to provide additional financing through such measures as cost recovery; reduction of the flight of the sector's resources and filling of vacant positions; improvement of the administration and management of the services; acceleration of the enactment of new laws and modification of existing ones regarding health care; restoration of the emphasis on primary health care, stressing maternal and child care and including family planning and disease control; improvement of the establishments and provision of additional services for mental patients, with modifications of the law to improve mental health services; reduction of the chronic deficit in drug supply in the health system; reorganization of the operation and administration of the General Department of Records; and collaboration with the private sector in health services delivery.

The collection of data for monitoring primary health care activities is accomplished through a monthly report that is analyzed at the central level.

In 1989, there were 18 general hospitals with 2708 beds, 5 specialized hospitals with 2319 beds, 1 maternity hospital with 229 beds, and 5 community hospitals that serve outpatients and normal deliveries, with 5 emergency beds each, which are occupied by the patients before their transfer to other hospitals. In 1987, there were 361 public health centers, 10 family planning clinics, 18 school dental clinics, and 6 mobile units.

In 1987, the country had 1.4 physicians, 0.2 dentists, 7.1 graduate nurses, 0.8 public health nurses, 3.6 nursing auxiliaries, 2.0 midwives, 2.2 community health auxiliaries, and 0.3 pharmacists per 10 000 population.

Public spending on health represented 2.9% of the GDP during 1989–1990. In 1988–1989, the Ministry of Health channeled 16.6% of its total spending into primary services.

Primary care

Primary care services are provided by 353 health centers, including 5 community hospitals that provide 24-hour service.

Primary care services are coordinated at the district, county, and regional levels by the District Medical Officer, the Medical Health Officer, and the Chief Health Officer, respectively, which facilitates the execution of the programs and enhances coordination.

Service delivery in the primary care centers is inadequate because of the shortage of human resources and supplies, the lack of suitable support services (transportation and communications), and scanty maintenance of the structure and equipment.

Several primary care activities are being carried out, including the construction and equipping of a public health laboratory; an information, education, and communication center for family planning; and several health centers; other health centers are being improved, as well. Progress also is being made in the process of decentralization.

Cooperation has been achieved with other public sectors, such as the Ministries of Labor and of Education; this cooperation is effective at the local level but has not been consolidated at the national level.

Health committees, which are the links between the Ministry of Health and the community, identify the health needs of their communities. Nongovernmental organizations participate in some health programs.

Jamaica receives support from other countries and from multilateral organizations for its health programs, and belongs to various regional health organizations.

It is estimated that approximately 80% of the population has access to the health services. In 1990, 67.4% of pregnant women were attended by qualified personnel and 18.4% of the total were seen prior to the sixteenth week of pregnancy; 70.4% of infants received adequate care. In 1989, 79% of deliveries were attended by trained personnel.

In 1990 immunization coverage among children under 1 year of age reached 98% for BCG, 86% for DPT, 87% for polio vaccine, and 74% for measle vaccine.

In 1989, 83.4% of the population was being supplied with water that had been treated and 11.3% was receiving untreated water; 94% of the inhabitants had adequate excreta disposal systems.

MEXICO

Demographic factors

The estimated population for 1990 was 88 598 000; however, the census carried out that year counted only 81 140 922 inhabitants. The annual growth rate for 1985–1990 was estimated at 2.2%. Of the total population, 35% is under 15 years of age. In 1987, 67% of the population lived in urban areas. The birthrate in 1987 was 34 per 1000 population and the fertility rate for 1985–1990 was estimated at 3.6 children per woman (the figure for 1986 was 3.8).

Socioeconomic factors

The per capita GDP in 1990 was US$2360 and the inflation rate for 1980–1989 was 72.7% per year.

The unemployment rate was estimated at between 15% and 18% in 1990; 12.7% of the population is illiterate.

Health indicators

Total mortality for 1987 was 4.9 per 1000 population and infant mortality was 31 per 1000 live births (for 1985–1990 it was estimated at 43 per 1000). Maternal mortality for 1987 was reported to be 5.6 per 10 000 live births.

Life expectancy at birth for 1985–1990 was 68.9 years.

The leading causes of mortality are diseases of the heart, accidents, malignant neoplasms, and intestinal infections.

Birthweight was known for approximately one-third of live births. Of these, 5% had a birthweight of under 2500 grams.

According to the National Nutrition Survey of 1988, 40% of the children under 5 years of age showed some degree of malnutrition (based on weight-for-age). According to the Waterlow scale, 66% of children under 5 years of age fell into the normal range, 15% were acutely malnourished, almost 12% had been malnourished but had subsequently recovered (low height-for-age with normal weight-for-height), and slightly more than 2% showed serious problems of acute chronic malnutrition.

Health care system

The health care system is made up of many institutions in the public sector plus those in the private sector.

The 1990–1994 National Health Plan consolidates the actions of the National Health System through the Ministry of Health. The Plan is governed by policies of health culture promotion; universal access to health services, with equity and quality; prevention and control of diseases and accidents; environmental protection and basic sanitation; contribution to population growth regulation; and promotion of social welfare. The strategies enunciated for this purpose are: functional coordination of the national health system; strengthening of local health systems; decentralization of health services; modernization and administrative streamlining; intersectoral coordination; and community participation. Among the priority projects to be developed are maternal and child health care; basic sanitation and environmental health; strengthening of decentralization of the health services toward the general population; and eradication and control of regional endemic diseases.

Decentralization has been initiated, and in 14 of the 31 federative entities it has been accomplished. At the different state and municipal levels, planning committees have been created, which have health and social security subcommittees whose purpose is to establish and evaluate programs.

The health services are accessible to 94% of the population, leaving a very scattered rural population group to be covered.

The financial resources allocated to the health sector represented 2.9% of the GDP in 1990. In 1989, 83.44% of public spending on the health sector was allocated to social security institutions and 16.56% to direct health care for the general population.

In 1990, the country had 3.89 physicians, 0.65 dentists, 7.2 nurses, and 9.4 nursing auxiliaries per 10 000 population.

Primary care

Primary care is delivered through rural health posts or clinics, auxiliary health units, mobile units, rural health centers for scattered populations, rural health centers for concentrated populations, and urban health centers. General hospitals, although their basic function is not primary care, carry out some activities in that area and provide support for the services. Community participation is being promoted and, as a specific line of action, community health committees have been created; between 1988 and 1990, the Mexican Social Security Institute (IMSS) created 1636. Health assemblies also are conducted in the communities covered by IMSS-Solidarity.

Activities have been carried out to train rural midwives as a way to improve deliveries in the communities.

In 1989, 50% of pregnant women were served by trained personnel, as were 68% of children; 45% of deliveries occurred in institutions. Currently, there is an effort to improve the information system.

In 1990, immunization coverage among children under 1 year of age was 70% for BCG, 66% for DPT, 96% for polio vaccine, and 78% for measles vaccine. In 1989, 39% of pregnant women received tetanus toxoid.

Water supply reached 68.71% of the total population (80.20% of the urban population and 40.65% of the rural); adequate excreta disposal was available to 45.18% of the total population (60.17% of the urban population and 8.57% of the rural).

NICARAGUA

Demographic factors

The total population in 1990 was estimated at 3.9 million, with an annual estimated growth rate of 3.4% for 1985–1990. Persons under 15 years of age made up 46% of the population. In 1990, it was estimated that 60% of the population was urban. The estimated birthrate for 1985–1990 was 42 per 1000 population and the fertility rate was 5.5 children per woman.

Socioeconomic factors

The rate of illiteracy, which was 12.8% in 1980, increased to 20% in 1990. The GDP per inhabitant in 1990 was estimated at US$470 and unemployment, at 35%. The annual inflation rate for the period from 1988 to 1990 was above 1000%.

Health indicators

For 1985–1990, total mortality was estimated at 8 per 1000 population and infant mortality, at 71 per 1000 live births.

Mortality among children aged 1–4 years was 9.6 per 1000.

Life expectancy at birth for 1985–1990 was estimated at 63.3 years.

The leading causes of death are diarrheal diseases, followed by diseases of the heart, cerebrovascular disease, and pneumonia.

Diarrhea and other infectious diseases account for a high percentage of the consultations at health services.

In 1986, 12% of newborns weighed under 2500 grams.

A height-for-age deficit was found in 22% of schoolchildren aged 6–9 years in 1980 and 18.7% in 1989. The prevalence of goiter among those 14 years of age was 3.9%, according to a survey carried out in 1989.

Health care system

The National Health System, which falls under the Ministry of Health, has functioned since the 1980s; it includes all public sector health services, including the medical services of social security. The health services are regionalized with three political-administrative levels: central, regional, and local. At the local level there are two administrative areas: the health area and the hospital.

The Constitution that went into effect in 1987 emphasizes the population's right to health.

The three-year plan for 1988–1990 established a health policy, the principal aims of which, according to the Ministry of Health, are:

—To reduce infant mortality, focusing on children under 1 year of age and on the rural and marginal urban areas.

—To reduce mortality and morbidity from violent causes and provide care for the disabled.

—To reduce morbidity and mortality from pesticides and other toxic substances, along with accidents and occupational risks.

—To reduce the incidence of sexually transmitted diseases, food poisoning, and alcoholism.

—To reduce the prevalence of malaria and its mortality.

—To reduce morbidity and mortality from typhoid fever, hepatitis, and tuberculosis.

—To reduce mortality from chronic and degenerative diseases and the prevalence of and trend toward chronicity in mental disorders.

In 1988, local health systems were defined as territorial health services, and in 1989, the municipal health services were established as a means of redirecting the reorganization of the first level of care. A local planning methodology also was developed, which made it possible to prepare the municipal health services programming mechanisms which were utilized in 1990 for these services' review and adjustment. It has been acknowledged that this level suffers from limitations regarding information that restrict the possibilities for planning at the municipal level.

Community participation has significantly supported the "Defense of the Life of the Child" campaign, enabling this effort to have an effect on other health areas.

The Ministry of Health's budget constituted 12.5% and 19% of the national budgets in 1989 and 1990, respectively. In the latter year, 45% was allotted for secondary care and 31% for primary care.

In 1987, there were 619 health units in operation: 30 hospitals (26 for acute care), 22 health centers with beds and 85 without beds, and 482 health posts.

In 1990, the Ministry of Health had 5.4 physicians, 0.67 dentists, 4.08 nurses, and 11.2 nursing auxiliaries per 10 000 population. There is considerable turnover among health personnel in the public sector, mainly owing to low pay.

Health technology primarily relies on imports. Efforts have been made to standardize technology acquisition, according to what the sector can absorb and maintain. Natural medicine and acupuncture have been promoted; medical professionals in the country have been studying the latter.

Primary care

Although 87% of pregnant women were reported to have received prenatal care in 1990, only 41.6% of all deliveries were attended in institutions; 71.9% of them also involved postnatal consultations (75.3% in 1989).

Monitoring of growth and development reached 97.3% of children under 1 year of age and 18.6% of children aged 1–5 years.

Immunization coverage among children under 1 year of age in 1989 and 1990 was, respectively, 92% and 81% for BCG, 68% and 65% for DPT, 85% and 86% for polio vaccine, and 63% and 82% for measles vaccine.

Oral rehydration units have significantly developed.

In 1988, drinking water services covered 53.23% of the total population (77.86% of the urban population and 18.9% of the rural); 18.91% of the total population and 32.48% of the urban population had sewerage services.

Regarding nutrition, a guide for the care of undernourished children at the hospital level began to be used; a program of continuing education was implemented; and the first draft of a manual on diets was prepared, along with the manuals for procedures, organization, policies, and standards for departments of nutrition and milk banks and laboratories. In addition, steps are being taken to reactivate the iodization of salt, and an intersectoral plan for the promotion of breast-feeding and a group feeding program at the hospital and community levels are being implemented.

Efforts also have been made to improve the sanitary control of food.

In the Ministry of Health an international cooperation unit has been created to promote and coordinate cooperation activities with bilateral, multilateral, and nongovernmental organizations. Financing that relies on international assistance has decreased from 0.81% of the total budget in 1985 to 0.20% and 0.21% in 1989 and 1990, respectively.

PANAMA

Demographic factors

The estimated population in 1990 was 2 814 000, 47% of it rural. The population is distributed over more than 9000 communities, of which some 7400 have fewer than 100 inhabitants. Persons under 15 years of age represent 35% of the population. For 1985–1990, the annual population growth rate was estimated at 2.07%, the birthrate at 26.7 per 1000 population, and the fertility rate at 3.1 children per woman.

Socioeconomic factors

The per capita GDP was US$1830 in 1990, and the inflation rate for 1980–1989 was 2.5% per year. The urban unemployment rate was 16.8% in 1990, and 11.9% of the population was illiterate. According to the Ministry of Planning and Economic Policy, 33.6% of the population was living in poverty in 1987.

Health indicators

The mortality rate remained at approximately 5.5 per 1000 population in the 1980s. Infant mortality was estimated at 23 per 1000 live births for 1985–1990 and was 22.8 in 1988. Reported maternal mortality was 6 per 10 000 live births.

Life expectancy at birth for 1985–1990 was 72 years.

The leading causes of death in 1988 were malignant neoplasms, external causes, cerebrovascular disease, and acute myocardial infarction.

The primary causes of morbidity in 1989 were diseases of the respiratory system and infectious and parasitic diseases.

Among children born in institutions, 8.1% weighed less than 2500 grams at birth, and it was reported that 24.4% of children suffer from some degree of malnutrition.

Health care system

The Constitution states that one of the State's duties is to safeguard health. There is effective coordination among the Ministry of Health, the Social Security Fund, and the Institute of Water Supply and Sewerage Systems. In 1990, new health policies were announced that emphasized, as part of the global strategy of primary care, the extension of coverage, environmental sanitation, nutrition, decentralization, health services management, comprehensive care, participation by the population, and coordination between and within sectors. The development and strengthening of local health systems are considered essential to the implementation of these policies. In addition, the need to narrow the health gap between different groups in the country has been stressed. The Health Code is being revised, in order to adapt it to the new needs.

The country is divided into 12 health regions, most of which correspond to the provincial divisions. Unfortunately, the process of decentralization has been slow and many decisions continue to be made at the central level.

Panama has 6 national, 13 regional, and 4 general hospitals; 15 rural or district hospitals; 26 health centers with beds and 114 without beds; 24 polyclinics without beds; 105 health subcenters; and 350 health posts.

In 1989, the country had 11.91 physicians, 2.14 dentists, 0.49 pharmacists, 10.56 nurses, 14.14 nursing auxiliaries, 0.68 dental assistants, 0.78 sanitation inspectors, 3.17 laboratory workers, 0.26 nutritionists, 0.18 health educators, and 0.46 social workers per 10 000 population.

In 1990, 9.96% of the GDP was spent on health; 11% of that was devoted to local services.

Primary care

Efforts are being made to increase the quality and coverage of primary care, but it is difficult to achieve broad coverage in rural areas because the population is so scattered. It is estimated that 99.9% and 61.9% of the urban and rural populations, respectively, have access to health services; the national average is 88.9%.

Community participation in health activities is being promoted and developed, and numerous nongovernmental organizations have been created for this purpose.

In 1990, 82.3% of pregnant women received care from qualified personnel (99.9% in urban areas and 64.7% in rural); 80.4% of children under 1 year of age also received such care (96% in urban areas and 64.8% in rural). Trained personnel attended 85.2% of deliveries (99.9% in urban areas and 70.5% in rural). Some contraceptive method is used by 58% of the women of childbearing age (86.4% and 28.6% of those in urban and rural areas, respectively).

Immunization coverage in 1990 reached 97% for BCG, 86% for DPT and polio vaccine, and 99% for measles vaccine.

In 1988, 82.65% of the population was being supplied with drinking water (100% of the urban population and 66.18% of the rural) and 83.65% (99.91% in urban areas and 68.23% in rural) had adequate excreta disposal systems.

Panama receives assistance from other countries and from international organizations and maintains agreements with neighboring countries for health activities.

PARAGUAY

Demographic factors

The estimated population for 1990 was 4 277 000. The annual growth rate for 1985–1990 was estimated at 2.93%. More than 30% of the inhabitants are concentrated in the city of Asunción and the Central Department, and 53% live in rural areas. In 1982, 42.4% of the population was under 15 years of age and 3.5% was 65 years old or older. The birthrate for 1980–1985 was estimated at 34.8 per 1000 population and the fertility rate, at 4.6 children per woman.

Socioeconomic factors

The per capita GDP in 1990 was US$1150 and the inflation rate averaged 23.2% per year from 1980 to 1989. In 1983, 22.5% of the population was illiterate, and in 1990, the urban unemployment rate was 6.6%.

Health indicators

Estimated total mortality for 1985–1990 was 6.6 per 1000 population; the figure reported for 1987 was 5.3. Infant mortality was estimated at 49 per 1000 live births for 1985–1990; for the last year in that period, it was recorded at 47.04. Registered maternal mortality has remained at 27.0 per 10 000 live births in recent years.

Life expectancy at birth was estimated at 66.9 years for 1985–1990.

The leading causes of death for 1980–1984 were diseases of the heart, cerebrovascular disease, malignant neoplasms, and acute respiratory diseases.

The leading reasons for consultation were acute respiratory diseases, diarrhea, and parasitic diseases.

Birthweights were under 2500 grams for 5.2% of the live births in 1990. In 1986, the prevalence of goiter in the population aged 6–15 years was 59.8%.

Health care system

The health sector's principal institutions are the Ministry of Public Health and Social Welfare, which is responsible for serving between 60% and 65% of the population and is the system's manager; the Institute of Social Welfare, which covers 14%; and the Health Department of the Armed Forces, which covers another 10%. The rest of the population is covered by the private sector and other minor public institutions. The Ministry follows a comprehensive-care policy, whereas the other institutions have an almost exclusively curative orientation.

Since 1989, new lines of action have been incorporated into the health policy—noteworthy among them are care for priority groups in accordance with the principles of social justice; strengthening of the managerial role of the Ministry and the participation of the other sectors; development of the operating capacity and functional articulation of the institutions of the sector; expansion of social security; definition of lines of action with regard to workers' health, elderly persons, and the participation of women in health and development; the development of closer ties with the countries of the Southern Cone; and initiation of the process of municipalization.

Among the actions aimed at achieving the aforementioned objectives are: the provision of free care to mothers and children and to those who have diseases with which the State is concerned (tuberculosis, Chagas' disease, malaria, and leprosy); intensification of vaccination activities; strengthening of nutrition programs; execution of the National Program for Human Development and Improvement of the Quality of Life, which is directed toward the population that lives in critical poverty, especially children in rural areas and women; formulation and implementation of the national plan for the Second Drinking Water Supply and Sanitation Decade; care for indigenous groups and people in new rural settlements; and the intensification of agricultural production.

In 1990, the Strategic Sectoral Plan for Health was formulated and its implementation was begun; it emphasizes the expansion of health care coverage, environmental control, strengthening primary care, control of the most prevalent diseases, development of comprehensive health care, and fostering community participation.

The National Health Council was created to improve the coordination of activities.

In terms of information, the available data in most of the health services, which have different systems and limited coordination, are incomplete and of limited use.

In 1990, 3.2% of the GDP was devoted to the health sector. The Ministry allotted 4.6% of its budget to health promotion and prevention activities, 6.6% to administration, and 88.8% to rehabilitation of health.

In 1989, there were 683 health institutions: 17 hospitals, 209 health centers, and 457 health posts. Of that total, 457 fell under the Ministry of Public Health and Social Welfare, and 120 under the Institute of Social Welfare. There was a total of 5437 beds available, of which 47.18% were located in the greater metropolitan area of Asunción.

In 1990, Paraguay had 7.00 physicians, 2.62 dentists, 0.81 nurses, 6.22 nursing auxiliaries, 2.05 midwives, 3.54 pharmacists, and 0.24 social workers per 10 000 population.

Primary care

The country has adopted the strategy of local health systems; this approach, along with decentralization, has been applied since 1990 as a mechanism for making health care more efficient.

Starting in 1989 the methodology of local planning has been incorporated in the institutions of the Ministry. Subnetworks to support diagnosis and treatment and for emergency care have been created, and the role of the hospitals has been defined.

The Ministry's Department of Social Welfare is formulating a policy for participation in health activities, and at all levels there is an effort to promote community involvement.

It is estimated that in 1990 approximately 60% of pregnant women, 60% of deliveries, and 64% of the children under 1 year of age received care from trained personnel. Tetanus toxoid was administered to 62.9% of pregnant women, and 44.1% of the women of childbearing age use some method of contraception.

Immunization coverage among children under 1 year old in 1990 was 90% for BCG, 78% for DPT, 76% for polio vaccine, and 69% for measles vaccine.

In 1988, 32.97% of the population had access to drinking water (64.97% in urban areas and 7.38% in rural) and 57.62% had adequate excreta disposal systems (54.65% in urban areas and 59.99% in rural).

Paraguay receives support from other countries and from multilateral organizations to carry out its activities, and has cooperative agreements with neighboring countries for the solution of common problems.

PERU

Demographic factors

The estimated population for 1990 was 22 332 000. The annual growth rate for 1985–1990 was estimated at 2.51%. The urban population comprises 70.2% of the total, and the city of Lima accounts for 31% of the country's population. In 1988, 39% of the population was under 15 years of age. The recorded birthrate was 32.2 per 1000 population, and the fertility rate for 1985–1990 was estimated at 4.5 children per woman.

Socioeconomic factors

The per capita GDP was US $1090 in 1990. The inflation rate for 1980–1989 was 160.3% per year. The rate of illiteracy was 14.9%. In 1989, the rate of unemployment for metropolitan Lima was 7.9% and the rate of underemployment was 73.8%.

Health indicators

Total mortality in 1989 was 9.4 per 1000 population; infant mortality was 88 per 1000 live births and maternal mortality, 24 per 10 000 live births.

Life expectancy at birth was 61.4 years for 1985–1990.

Diseases of the heart constitute the leading cause of death; diseases of the respiratory system also are significant causes. Tuberculosis is among the ten leading causes of death and is a significant factor in morbidity.

Infectious and parasitic diseases are the predominant causes of morbidity. Malaria is also a significant problem, since 74% of the country has ecological conditions favorable for its transmission. Goiter constitutes a serious problem: 90% of the rural populations in the mountains and 75% of those along the coast live in areas where this disease is endemic. Its prevalence in schoolchildren is 38% in the mountains and 21% along the coast; however, populations with prevalences of up to 90% in that age group have been identified.

The percentage of children with birthweight under 2500 grams is 7.5%. It is reported that of children under 6 years of age 62% in the rural areas and 15% in the urban areas show some degree of malnutrition.

Health care system

The health care system is made up of many services in the public and private sectors. In the public sector the major organizations are the Ministry of Health and the Peruvian Social Security Institute (IPSS).

Health policy for 1985–1990 had as its central objective the democratization of health. This policy was supported by a set of guidelines that included mobilization and participation of the people, decentralization of the health services, multisectoral action, development of new approaches and technologies to address the health problems, and adaptation of the health sector and its institutions to the new policy and to the leading role of the Ministry of Health in the formulation and application of the policies.

For 1990–1995, the objectives that have been set are: defense of the life and health of Peruvians, the democratization of health, and the reconstruction and renewal of the health sector as an instrument for the development of social policy. The specific policies are comprehensive health, health as the responsibility of all, decentralization and regionalization, prioritization of the local level upgrading of human resources, scientific development and technological production, drugs as a social good, restoration of the health establishments, reorientation of the IPSS, and reorientation of technical cooperation.

The following strategies for implementing the policy have been established: extension activities and social mobilization for health, social consensus-building, the strengthening of the leadership role of the Ministry, intensification of the process of decentralization, reorientation of health actions, and emphasis on labor conditions in the sector.

In 1988, the National Health Council was established as an advisory body under the Ministry and the installation of the Regional Councils was initiated (by 1991, 12 of the 14 planned Councils had been established). In four departments, the functional integration of the Ministry and the IPSS has been initiated, but only in the hospitals. The transfer of the health services managed by the Ministry to the operational levels has been initiated. Through this process, responsibility is transferred from the first level of care to the municipalities, which also are responsible for water supply and basic sanitation. The second and third levels of care will be the responsibility of the regional level, and the central government will be responsible for specialized services at the fourth level of care.

Rather than being regionalized, IPSS is being decentralized by naming directors in the regions.

Spending on health represented 3.4% of the GDP in 1989.

In 1990, there were 368 hospitals with 34 432 beds (1.5 per 1000 population), 1020 health centers with beds (75% in the Ministry of Health), and 3174 health posts (94% in the Ministry).

For the same year, the country had 10.2 physicians, 2.4 dentists, 7.9 nurses, 2.8 pharmacists, and 1.7 midwives per 10 000 population. Of the physicians, 59% were in institutions at the third and fourth levels, 23% at the second level, and 18% at the first level.

Primary care

The country's priority health programs aim at child survival, control of acute diarrheal diseases, control of acute respiratory infections, immunization, growth and development, family planning, control of tuberculosis, control of goiter and cretinism, and control of malaria.

The importance of community participation has been acknowledged, and the Bureau of Support for Community Participation and Mobilization was created within the Ministry to encourage more participation from the community. In addition, mothers' clubs and community kits of essential drugs administered by the community itself were created, and between 1985 and 1990 some 10 000 health workers were trained.

Recently, the coverage of health services in rural and marginal urban areas has been expanded through the creation of new posts for professionals from the various disciplines.

It was reported that for 1985–1990 only 8% of the women of childbearing age used any method of contraception.

In 1990, immunization coverage among children under 1 year of age reached 83% for BCG, 72% for DPT, 73% for polio vaccine, and 64% for measles vaccine.

In 1988, 58.44% of the population was supplied with drinking water (77.60% of the urban population and 22.31% of the rural) and 41.70% had adequate excreta disposal services (55.00% of the urban population and 16.60% of the rural).

SURINAME

Demographic factors

The population in 1990 was estimated at 422 000. The growth rate for 1985–1990 was 1.94% per year. One-half the population lives in rural areas. Persons under 15 years of age constitute 36%. The birthrate registered in 1987 was 24.6 per 1000 population and the fertility rate for 1985–1990 was estimated at 2.97 children per woman.

Socioeconomic factors

The per capita GDP in 1989 was US$3020. In 1990, the urban unemployment rate was 33%, and the illiteracy rate was 15.5% for men and 23.8% for women.

Health indicators

Estimated total mortality for 1981–1986 was 7 per 1000 population per year. Infant mortality for 1985–1990 was estimated at 31 per 1000 live births per year; in 1988 it was registered at 24.6 per 1000. Maternal mortality in 1987 was 3.1 per 10 000 live births; mortality among children aged 1–4 years was 1.8 per 1000.

Life expectancy at birth for 1985–1990 was 69.5 years.

In 1980, 13% of the children born in hospitals (50% of all births) weighed less than 2500 grams. Through monitoring services it was determined that from 8% to 18% of children aged 0–5 years were below the third percentile for weight-for-age.

The leading causes of death are ischemic heart disease, perinatal causes, malignant neoplasms, accidents, cerebrovascular disease, influenza, suicides, diarrhea, diabetes, asthma, and bronchitis.

The leading causes of morbidity are diabetes and influenza, followed by gastroenteritis, sexually transmitted diseases, and accidents. In a study of 1986–1987 it was estimated that 2.7% of the population had some form of disability—in 47.5% of these cases, the disability was due to mental causes; in 44.6%, physical problems; and in 8%, chronic diseases.

Health care system

The health sector includes, in addition to the Ministry of Health, many semipublic foundations that technically depend on the Ministry of Health and are financed with public funds. It also includes the private sector. Health services are provided through hospitals, clinics, and health posts.

The health policy has placed new emphasis on the development of local health systems and community participation, as well as on the strengthening of financial control of the health sector. The policy set by the government in 1990 gave priority to the areas of management; epidemiological surveillance; physical infrastructure and supplies; protection of especially vulnerable groups; disease control, including zoonotic diseases; environmental health; and human resources development.

The Regional Health Service, a nongovernmental organization that has existed since 1990, provides basic primary care services on the coastal plain through health centers and primary care offices and clinics. Health care in the interior is the responsibility of the Medical Mission, which is a private institution.

Epidemiological surveillance has improved and has become more timely through a national surveillance system with sentinel stations and telephone communications; epidemiological surveillance of the nutritional status of children under 5 years old, schoolchildren, and refugees has been added. The malaria and vector control situations also are monitored, and there is a committee to monitor the health system.

There is no national policy regarding the selection of health technology. There is a proposal to form a research council that would develop a health research program for the country. An inventory of the research projects under way in the area of health is being prepared.

In 1990, the country had 1892 hospital beds, and in 1989 there were 9 hospitals (3 public and 6 private), 12 health centers, 32 Ministry of Health medical offices, and 91 clinics.

In 1990, there were 8.04 physicians, 0.79 dentists, 1.76 dental nurses, and 0.50 pharmacists per 10 000 population; and in 1991, 18.78 nurses, 8.55 nursing assistants, 3.86 nursing auxiliaries, and 1.34 midwives per 10 000 population. There is a concentration of resources in the capital, although it has become less pronounced in recent years.

In 1990, government spending on health constituted 5.7% of the GDP and, in 1989, 16% of the budget was devoted to primary care.

Primary care

Primary care services are provided by the Regional Health Service and the Medical Mission. There are difficulties in the acceptance of primary care because of the way in which physicians and nurses are educated and a curriculum that is not adapted to the realities of primary care. There is good functional intersectoral collaboration, especially with the Ministries of Education, of Agriculture, of Public Works, of Regional Development, of Social Affairs, and of Economic Affairs and with the Central Planning Office.

Steps have been taken to decentralize the process of decision-making; however, this has not been fully accomplished. Many nongovernmental organizations participate in health activities. Preparations are being made to mount a national education campaign on lifestyles in order to raise the public's awareness of the importance of its contribution to its own health, as well as the importance of participation in developing the community's health.

Suriname receives assistance for its health programs from several countries, particularly from the Netherlands and Belgium, and from international organizations. In addition, it participates in programs with neighboring countries.

It was estimated that 95% of the urban population and 90% of the rural population had access to health services in 1990. Specialized personnel attended 98% of the deliveries.

In a sample of 550 women of childbearing age interviewed in 1990, it was found that 54.7% were using some method of contraception.

In 1990, immunization coverage among children under 1 year was 83% for DPT, 81% for polio vaccine, and 65% for measles vaccine.

In 1988, 71.90% of the total population had drinking water (78.04% of the urban population and 53.54% of the rural) and 55.95% had adequate excreta disposal systems (63.18% of the urban population and 34.34% of the rural).

TRINIDAD AND TOBAGO

Demographic factors

The population in 1990 was estimated at 1 160 000 and the growth rate for 1985–1990 was 1.3% per year. Approximately 30% of the population lives in rural areas. In the 1980s, 33.2% of the population was under 15 years of age, and 5.7% was 65 or older. The birthrate in 1986 was estimated at 27 per 1000 population and the fertility rate for 1985–1990, at 2.95 children per woman.

Socioeconomic factors

The per capita GDP in 1989 was US$3230 and the annual inflation rate for 1980–1989 was 5.8%.

The illiteracy rate in 1990 was 7.2% and the unemployment rate was estimated at 20%. At the end of 1988, an estimated 18% of the population was living in poverty.

Health indicators

Total mortality in 1989 was 6.6 per 1000 population and infant mortality for 1985–1990 was estimated at 24 per 1000 live births. Maternal mortality in 1989 was 8 per 10 000 births.

Life expectancy at birth for 1985–1990 was estimated at 70.2 years.

The leading causes of death are diseases of the heart, followed by malignant neoplasms, cerebrovascular disease, diabetes mellitus, pneumonia, and accidents.

In 1988, birthweights for 13% of the live births were under 2500 grams.

A survey carried out in 1987 revealed that among children under 3 years of age, the prevalence of protein-energy malnutrition was 7.6% for girls and 6.2% for boys, and that the prevalence of severe malnutrition, based on weight-for-height, was 3.9% for girls and 3.8% for boys.

Health care system

The health care system, traditionally of a public-assistance type, is shifting to a mixed model that includes privatization, national health insurance, and regionalization. However, most health care continues to be provided by the Ministry of Health.

The Government approved the Macroeconomic Framework for National Reconstruction, 1989–1995, which sets out the policy, strategies, and programs proposed for the development of all sectors, including the health sector. This framework endorses the idea of primary care and recognizes the importance of the measures to be taken in order to ensure the well-being of the nation. In order to coordinate the execution of agreed measures, a national planning committee was established, along with various subcommittees.

The principal objectives of the established policy involve stressing the importance of lifestyles and habits in the population, promoting and maintaining an adequate program of educational activities, making health services available to the population at a reasonable cost, ensuring that the basic health services are within the reach of all sectors of the population, reducing the incidence of environmental health problems, promoting strict health standards and industrial safety, and promoting intersectoral coordination in health services delivery.

The Government has proposed a national system of health insurance that will increase access to private care and ensure universal coverage; the Government would assume responsibility for the indigent and low-income segments of the population.

Actions to decentralize and regionalize the Ministry of Health services were being initiated, and the process of establishing a central unit that will be responsible for managing the health information system has begun.

In 1991, the health sector accounted for 2.6% of the GDP. In 1990, 9.07% of the Ministry's budget was devoted to local services.

In 1989, the country had two general, four district, and two county hospitals, three specialized hospitals (mental, rehabilitation, and geriatric), and four extended-care facilities. There were, in addition, two maternity hospitals and seven delivery units attached to health centers. There were also over 100 primary-level health care centers in strategic locations.

In 1986 there were 9.20 physicians, 1.08 dentists, 27.89 nurses (including midwives), 1.09 public health inspectors, 0.38 social workers, and 2.14 public health nurses per 10 000 population. Training courses are provided for all the workers in the health sector. Medical interns must perform community service for three months as a part of their training.

Primary care

Primary care services are administered by the Principal Medical Officer. These community services are administratively divided into nine counties, each under a medical officer who supervises the health personnel in each area.

In order to improve primary care, the Government has proposed channeling more resources into this area; committing more resources for health education activities; shifting to a decentralized structure; concentrating on high-risk groups such as mothers and children, hypertensives, diabetics, and the elderly; formulating a national nutrition plan; redesigning the oral health program; and initiating multidisciplinary research.

The mechanisms for patient referral have improved little in recent years, but it is hoped that this will change with decentralization.

Several nongovernmental organizations are involved in health-related activities. Community leaders attend some meetings of the National Planning Committee to express their points of view.

In 1990, it was estimated that 99% of the population had access to the health services and that almost all pregnant women and all infants were served by trained personnel. In 1988, 98% of deliveries were attended by trained personnel.

In 1987, 53% of women of childbearing age were using some contraceptive method.

In 1990, immunization coverage among children under 1 year of age was 82% for DPT, 87% for polio vaccine, and 70% for measles vaccine.

In 1988, 95.93% of the total population had access to drinking water (100% of the urban population and 87.17% of the rural) and 99.19% had adequate excreta disposal systems (97.44% of the rural population).

The country receives international assistance from other countries and from multilateral organizations, especially for personnel training and medical treatments.

THE UNITED STATES OF AMERICA

Demographic factors

The population in 1990 was estimated at 249 235 000. During 1985–1990 the annual growth rate was 0.81%. Rural inhabitants account for 25.95% of the population. The birthrate in 1988 was 15.9 per 1000 population and the fertility rate for 1985–1990 was 1.8 children per woman.

Socioeconomic factors

The per capita GDP for 1988–1989 was US$21 000, and the annual inflation rate for 1980–1989 was 4.0%. The illiteracy rate is estimated at 0.5% in the population over 15 years of age. In 1990, the rate of urban unemployment reached 8.8%.

Health indicators

In 1988, infant mortality was 10.0 per 1000 live births (8.5 for whites and 17.6 for blacks). For the same year, maternal mortality was 0.84 per 10 000 births; in 1989 it was 0.7.

Life expectancy at birth for 1985–1990 was 75.4 years. Of the children born in 1988, 6.9% weighed under 2500 grams, (5.6% for whites, 13% for blacks, and 11.5% for other races).

In 1968, the five leading causes of death were diseases of the heart, malignant neoplasms, cerebrovascular diseases, accidents and other violence, and chronic obstructive pulmonary disease.

In 1989, the most important causes of morbidity were hypertension, auditory disorders, alcoholism, diseases of the heart, diabetes, accidents and other violence, human immunodeficiency virus infection, malignant tumors, and cerebrovascular disease. It was estimated that 14.1% of the population has some kind of physical limitation, and 9.6% were restricted in their principal activity because of a chronic disease.

Health care system

The health care system combines public and private services; the private sector accounts for most health spending.

The Federal Government's main health agency—the Department of Health and Human Services—develops national health policies and objectives and coordinates the work of its multiple agencies in order to support those policies and objectives. The Department administers a broad network of health programs, among them the financing of health care for the elderly and the poor; the prevention, diagnosis, and treatment of some diseases through basic and epidemiological research; and the delivery of health services to special groups, directly or by providing incentives for this purpose. In addition, it serves as a central point for health services research.

The goals set for the year 2000 are to increase the length of healthy life for the population, to reduce the disparities in health, and to achieve access to preventive services for all. On this basis 300 quantifiable objectives have been set; they are grouped into 22 priority areas, which fall into the following three categories:

—Health promotion, directed toward individual or community initiatives to reduce risks.
—Health protection, which includes aspects that can be modified by environmental or regulatory measures.
—Preventive services, which involve activities administered particularly in a clinical environment.

According to the data for 1987, almost one-half of the objectives had been achieved or it was very probable that they would be before 1990. Of the remaining objectives, there was little likelihood that 25% of them would be achieved; and there was no available data for evaluating the other 25%.

Some of the country's states have begun to set their own objectives in accordance with the national objectives. The state health departments will provide leadership to give prevention the highest priority, and they will encourage the communities to establish programs to reach the objectives.

In the United States health research is of paramount importance. Research priorities are set by combining scientific considerations with policy factors, such as the magnitude of the problem; the state of knowledge; the availability of personnel, facilities, and equipment; and the opinions of interested groups.

In 1986, the country had 6035 short-stay hospitals (1863 public) and 1 066 611 beds.

In 1987, there were 22.3 physicians, 5.8 dentists, 66.9 nurses, 6.4 pharmacists, 1.0 optometrists, and 1.9 veterinarians per 10 000 population. Even with this high rate, problems of accessibility, cost, and quality of care persist for large segments of the population.

To ensure the quality of care, in 1986 the law established the creation of a database containing information on problems encountered by physicians, dentists, and other health care providers in their practices.

In 1987, spending on health represented 11.2% of the GDP and personal health care accounted for 88% of that spending.

Primary care

Primary care services are available from private physicians and in community clinics. Although the value of primary care is well understood and accepted, this level is often not an individual's first point of contact with the health system. There are federal programs to ensure primary care for people who live in areas with limited medical services and those with special health needs, including the homeless and pregnant women.

There is extensive cooperation among various sectors to achieve the health objectives that have been set. In addition, there are formal channels of communication with the community designed to elicit its participation. Varying organizations participate in primary care programs.

The country provides assistance in health to other countries, and has signed bilateral agreements with some of them for research and for solving problems.

Most of the population has access to health services. In 1988, 98.3% of pregnant women whose pregnancies ended in a live birth received prenatal care from trained personnel, and 76.5% received care in the first trimester of pregnancy. With respect to deliveries, 99.1% occurred in hospitals and 99.3% were attended by trained personnel (95.9% by physicians and 3.4% by midwives). Almost all children receive care from trained personnel. Of the women between 15 and 44 years of age, 60% use some method of contraception.

According to some surveys, at least 85% of the women aged 15–45 are protected against tetanus. BCG vaccine is not administered. It is estimated that 70%–80% of children under 2 years of age are vaccinated against measles, rubella, diphtheria, poliomyelitis, tetanus, whooping cough, and mumps, and that approximately 85% of those under 6 months of age have received polio and DPT vaccines. The basic immunizations are compulsory for entry into day care centers, kindergarten, and primary school.

Nearly 90% of the population has access to potable water.

URUGUAY

Demographic factors

The estimated population in 1990 was 3 128 000; 85.46% was urban, 44% was concentrated in the Department of Montevideo, and the remainder were living in inland areas. The annual growth rate for 1985–1990 was estimated at 0.76%. A total of 26% of the population is under 15 years of age and 13% is 65 or older. The birthrate in 1989 was reported to be 18.1 per 1000 population and the fertility rate for 1985–1990 was estimated at 2.4 children per woman.

Socioeconomic factors

The per capita GDP in 1990 was US$2620, and the inflation rate for 1980–1989 was 59.2%. The rate of illiteracy in 1990 was 3.8%, and the urban unemployment rate was 9.3%.

Health indicators

Mortality has remained at approximately 10 per 1000 population since 1950. Infant mortality in 1989 was 21 per 1000 live births; for 1985–1990 it was estimated at 24 per 1000. Maternal mortality in 1989 was 2.5 per 10 000 live births.

Life expectancy at birth was 72.0 years for 1985–1990.

The leading causes of death are diseases of the circulatory system, malignant neoplasms, accidents, respiratory infections, and diabetes mellitus.

In 1986, 7.6% of newborns had birthweights under 2500 grams.

Health care system

The public sector of the health system is made up of the Ministry of Public Health, the Social Security Administration, and other medical services under the Ministries of the Interior and National Defense, the national university, municipal governments, and autonomous entities and decentralized services. The private sector includes institutions for collective medical care (IAMC) and sanatoriums, convalescent homes, and non-institutional private care facilities. In 1988 it was estimated that IAMCs covered 50.5% of the population; the rest of the private sector, 9.5%; the Ministry of Health and the University, 28.5%; the

Armed Forces, 10.5%; and other public institutions, 1.0%.

Currently there is no health information system that covers all the needs.

The Ministry of Health has 90 polyclinics and 21 health centers, which constitute the first level of care; 17 Type A and 13 Type B hospitals, which constitute the second level; 15 Type C hospitals, which usually cover a department and constitute the third level of complexity; and four Type D hospitals and 12 specialized institutes, which constitute the fourth level of care and cover the entire nation.

It is estimated that 6.51% of the GDP is spent on health.

In 1989, the country had 27.42 physicians and 4.8 graduate nurses per 10 000 population (of these, only 26.8% were employed professionally).

Primary health care

The Ministry of Health is committed to implementing the strategy of primary care; to this end, it has defined the following lines of action:

—Reorientation of health personnel toward primary care through regional workshops for primary-level personnel, the training of family doctors, and the publication of a magazine aimed at personnel at the operational level.

—Community participation in the planning, organization, and execution of primary care through activities in health education and personnel training.

—Intersectoral coordination through agreements with other institutions and the creation of departmental health committees.

—Normative centralization and executive decentralization.

—Interinstitutional coordination of health services that operate at the primary level of care, through agreements signed between some municipal governments and the Ministry.

—Application of the risk approach, with emphasis on maternal and child health programs.

—Coordination of teaching and service with the Schools of Medicine and Dentistry, and introduction of curriculum changes in the Ministry's School of Health.

—International cooperation, for which agreements with various institutions have been signed to provide support for primary care programs.

Community participation has been emphasized with the creation of the Division of Health Education within the Ministry of Health; this Division has prepared and disseminated information and has trained Ministry personnel, as well as taught intermediate-level personnel within other governmental and nongovernmental institutions.

The entire population has easy access to health services. In 1989, the proportion of pregnant women served by the public sector was 61.0% for Montevideo and 55.6% for the interior of the country; 42.0% and 37.7%, respectively, were seen in the first trimester. The private mutual insurance sector served 77.95% of pregnant women affiliated with it. Trained personnel attended 99.8% of deliveries.

In 1990, immunization coverage among children under 1 year of age was 99% for BCG, 88% for DPT and polio vaccines, and 82% for measles vaccine.

In 1988, drinking water services covered 84.92% of the population (96.62% of the urban population and 5.21% of the rural) and 60.40% had adequate excreta disposal systems (59.65% in urban areas and 65.36% in rural).

VENEZUELA

Demographic factors

The estimated population in 1990 was 19 736 000. The annual growth rate for 1985–1990 was 2.61%. The population is highly concentrated in 6 of the 23 Federal Entities, and 16.4% resides in rural areas. A total of 38.5% of the population is under 15 years of age and 3.6% is 65 years old or older. The birthrate in 1989 was 25.7 per 1000 population, and the fertility rate for 1985–1990 was 3.8 children per woman.

Socioeconomic factors

The per capita GDP was US$2420 in 1990. The annual rate of inflation for 1980–1989 was 16.0%. Unemployment reached 9.6% in the second half of 1989. It is estimated that 43.2% of the population lives at the poverty level. In 1990, the illiteracy rate was an estimated 11.9%.

Health indicators

In 1988, total mortality was 4.4 per 1000 population; infant mortality was 22.7 per 1000 live births; and maternal mortality was 6.0 per 10 000 live births.

Life expectancy at birth for 1985–1990 was 69.7 years.

Among those under 15 years of age examined in public health service facilities, 12.0% showed a slight height-for-age deficit; 3.4%, a moderate deficit; and 30%, a severe deficit.

The leading causes of death for all ages are diseases of the heart, malignant neoplasms, accidents, certain conditions originating in the perinatal period, and cerebrovascular disease. In children under 1 year of age the leading causes of death are: hypoxia, asphyxiation, and other respiratory diseases; enteritis and other diarrheal diseases; congenital anomalies; other conditions of the newborn; and diseases of the respiratory system.

In 1990, the leading reasons for consultation for children aged 5 years and older were colds, diarrhea, and pharyngoamygdalitis, and in children under 5, helminthiasis and mild respiratory infections.

Health care system

The health sector is made up of public and private subsectors. The public subsector consists of various institutions: the primary ones (based on the size of their investments and the population they cover) are the Ministry of Health and Social Welfare, the Venezuelan Social Security Institute, the Institute of Social Welfare within the Ministry of Education, and the Bureau of Health of the Federal District.

In 1987, the Organic Law of the National Health System was enacted. This law provides for the integration, under the direction and administration of the National Branch through the Ministry of Health and Social Welfare, of all the services devoted to safeguarding health in the country, and it also sets standards for the regulation of the activities of the private subsector. The integration of the public sector services will be completed over a period of 10 years, beginning from the date on which the Law went into effect.

The health sector's policy aims at increasing regionalization and decentralization of the health care services with normative centralization, achievement of progressive integration of all public health institutions in a single entity, and development of the programs for primary care, with emphasis on programs for health promotion and prevention of health problems and administrative reorganization of the sector. In addition, efforts are being made to develop a drug supply policy that will result in the provision of high-quality drugs at low cost to groups with limited resources.

In 1988, Venezuela had 386 Type I, 68 Type II, and 24 Type III urban outpatient clinics and 2489 Type I and 616 Type II rural clinics (not staffed by a physician but by an aide with basic medical training). In 1990, the country had 576 hospitals (266 public) and 55 662 hospital beds (2.6 per 1000 population).

In the same year, the country had 16.3 physicians, 7.7 nurses, 21.3 nursing auxiliaries, and 3.8 dentists per 1000 population. The distribution of human resources is uneven, with greater concentration in the most highly developed and populated states.

In 1985, spending on health in the public sector represented 1.8% of the GDP.

Primary care

Primary care services are provided in both urban and rural clinics. The Expanded Maternal and Child Health Program has been implemented with a view to improving health indicators and nutritional status among low-income women and children. The program aims at the sector of the population that is below the poverty line. It provides prenatal and postnatal care for mothers and monitoring of growth and development for children under 6 years of age.

Intersectoral coordination in health is still limited, although efforts are being undertaken to increase it.

Community and nongovernmental organizations participate in health programs, but their participation in programming is limited.

In 1989, 82% of deliveries were attended in institutions. Some contraceptive method is used by 14% of women of childbearing age.

In 1990, immunization coverage among children under 1 year of age was 63% for BCG and DPT, 72% for polio vaccine, and 62% for measles vaccine.

In 1988, 89.33% of the population had drinking water (89.44% of the urban population and 84.40% of the rural) and 92.39% had an adequate excreta disposal system (96.90% of the urban population and 70.09% of the rural).

ANNEX

Table 1. Estimated and projected population and annual geometric growth rates, by subregion and country, 1985, 1990, 1995, and 2000.

Subregion and country	Population (thousands)				Annual growth rates (percent)		
	1985	1990	1995	2000	1985–1990	1990–1995	1995–2000
Regional total	668 369	723 923	779 639	834 468	1.60	1.48	1.36
Latin America	396 681	440 631	485 817	531 194	2.10	1.95	1.79
Andean Area	81 477	91 983	103 010	114 329	2.43	2.26	2.09
Bolivia	6371	7314	8421	9724	2.76	2.82	2.88
Colombia	28 713	31 819	34 939	37 998	2.05	1.87	1.68
Ecuador	9378	10 782	12 314	13 939	2.79	2.66	2.48
Peru	19 698	22 332	25 123	27 952	2.51	2.36	2.13
Venezuela	17 317	19 736	22 213	24 716	2.61	2.37	2.14
Southern Cone	49 159	52 902	56 642	60 414	1.47	1.37	1.29
Argentina	30 331	32 322	34 264	36 238	1.27	1.17	1.12
Chile	12 121	13 173	14 237	15 272	1.66	1.55	1.40
Falkland Islands	2	2	2	2	0.0	0.0	0.0
Paraguay	3693	4277	4893	5538	2.93	2.69	2.48
Uruguay	3012	3128	3246	3364	0.76	0.74	0.71
Brazil	135 564	150 368	165 083	179 487	2.07	1.87	1.67
Central American Isthmus	25 370	29 073	33 306	37 892	2.72	2.72	2.58
Belize	163	182	201	221	2.19	2.02	1.85
Costa Rica	2642	3015	3374	3711	2.64	2.25	1.90
El Salvador	4767	5252	5943	6739	1.93	2.47	2.51
Guatemala	7963	9197	10 621	12 221	2.88	2.88	2.81
Honduras	4383	5138	5968	6846	3.18	3.00	2.74
Nicaragua	3272	3871	4540	5261	3.36	3.19	2.95
Panama	2180	2418	2659	2893	2.07	1.90	1.69
Mexico	79 376	88 598	97 967	107 233	2.20	2.01	1.81
Latin Caribbean	25 735	27 707	29 809	31 839	1.48	1.46	1.32
Cuba	9946	10 324	10 788	11 189	0.75	0.88	0.73
Haiti	5922	6504	7148	7837	1.88	1.89	1.84
Puerto Rico	3451	3709	3958	4192	1.44	1.30	1.15
Dominican Republic	6416	7170	7915	8621	2.22	1.98	1.71
Caribbean	6964	7468	7985	8504	1.40	1.34	1.26
Anguilla	7	7	8	8	1.42	1.32	1.24
Antigua and Barbuda	81	86	93	99	1.39	1.37	1.32
Bahamas	242	260	278	297	1.41	1.34	1.33
Barbados	253	261	272	285	0.62	0.82	0.96
Cayman Islands	20	21	23	24	1.45	1.27	1.36
Dominica	76	81	87	93	1.32	1.33	1.38
French Guiana	82	92	102	112	2.25	2.06	1.87
Grenada	96	103	110	117	1.33	1.33	1.38
Guadeloupe	334	340	346	354	0.34	0.37	0.45
Guyana	953	1040	1119	1197	1.74	1.46	1.34
Jamaica	2336	2521	2706	2886	1.52	1.41	1.29
Martinique	328	331	338	352	0.18	0.43	0.82
Netherlands Antilles	180	193	207	221	1.41	1.35	1.32
Turks and Caicos Islands	8	9	9	10	1.46	1.36	1.28
Virgin Islands (U.K.)	13	14	15	16	1.36	1.41	1.32
Virgin Islands (U.S.)	105	113	121	129	1.40	1.36	1.32
Montserrat	12	13	14	15	1.47	1.22	1.43
Saint Kitts and Nevis	46	50	53	57	1.41	1.32	1.34
Saint Vincent and the Grenadines	104	111	118	127	1.33	1.34	1.36
Saint Lucia	128	136	146	156	1.32	1.34	1.37
Suriname	375	403	435	469	1.46	1.52	1.49
Trinidad and Tobago	1185	1283	1385	1480	1.59	1.53	1.32
North America	264 724	275 824	285 837	294 770	0.82	0.71	0.62
Bermuda	56	58	60	62	0.70	0.70	0.70
Canada	25 379	26 525	27 567	28 508	0.88	0.77	0.67
United States	239 283	249 235	258 204	266 194	0.81	0.71	0.61
Saint Pierre and Miquelon	6	6	6	6	0.0	0.0	0.0

Source: United Nations. *World Population Prospect: 1988.* New York, 1989.

111

Table 2. Life expectancy at birth, by subregions, groups, and countries, 1950-2000.

Subregions, groups, and countries	Life expectancy at birth			Quinquennial increase		Life expectancy at birth	Population in 1990	
	1950–1955	1970–1975	1985–1990	1950–1955 to 1970–1975	1970–1975 to 1985–1990	Year 2000	Millions	Percentage
Latin America	51.8	61.2	66.6	2.4	1.8	69.7	438.0	100.0
1. Bolivia	40.4	46.7	53.1	1.6	2.1	60.5	7.3	
Haiti	37.6	48.5	54.7	2.7	2.1	59.4	6.5	
Total							13.8	3.2
2. Peru	43.9	55.5	61.4	2.9	2.0	67.9	22.3	
Guatemala	42.1	54.0	62.0	3.0	2.7	68.1	9.2	
El Salvador	45.3	58.8	62.2	3.4	1.1	68.8	5.3	
Nicaragua	42.3	54.7	63.3	3.1	2.9	69.3	3.9	
Honduras	42.3	54.0	64.0	2.9	3.3	68.2	5.1	
Total							45.8	10.5
3. Brazil	51.0	59.8	64.9	2.2	1.7	68.0	150.4	
Ecuador	48.4	58.9	65.4	2.6	2.2	68.2	10.6	
Dominican Republic	46.0	59.9	65.9	3.5	2.0	69.7	7.2	
Paraguay	62.6	65.6	66.9	0.7	0.4	67.9	4.3	
Colombia	50.6	61.6	68.2	2.8	2.2	70.7	33.0	
Mexico	50.8	62.6	68.9	3.0	2.1	72.1	88.6	
Venezuela	55.2	66.2	69.7	2.8	1.1	71.3	19.7	
Total							313.8	71.6
4. Argentina	62.7	67.3	70.6	1.1	1.1	72.3	32.3	
Chile	53.8	63.6	71.5	2.5	2.6	72.7	13.2	
Uruguay	66.3	68.8	72.0	0.6	1.1	73.0	3.1	
Panama	55.3	66.3	72.1	2.8	1.9	73.5	2.4	
Total							51.0	11.6
5. Costa Rica	57.3	68.1	74.7	2.7	2.2	75.8	3.0	
Cuba	59.5	71.0	75.2	2.9	1.4	76.3	10.6	
Total							13.6	3.1
Non-Latin Caribbean	56.4	67.1	72.4	2.7	1.8	74.7	6.2	100.0
1. Suriname	56.0	64.9	69.5	2.2	1.5	72.6	0.4	
Guyana	55.2	64.1	69.7	2.2	1.9	72.8	1.0	
Trinidad and Tobago	57.9	66.5	70.2	2.2	1.2	73.1	1.3	
Total							2.7	44.1
2. Guadeloupe	56.5	67.8	73.3	2.8	1.8	75.7	0.3	
Barbados	57.2	69.4	73.9	3.1	1.5	76.2	0.3	
Jamaica	57.2	67.8	74.0	2.6	2.1	76.2	2.5	
Martinique	56.5	68.8	74.2	3.1	1.8	76.4	0.3	
Total							3.5	55.9
North America	69.1	72.2	76.1	0.8	1.3	78.1	275.7	100.0
United States of America	69.0	71.3	75.4	0.6	1.4	77.6	249.2	
Canada	69.1	73.1	76.7	1.0	1.2	78.5	26.5	

Source: CELADE, 1990, and United Nations, 1989.

Table 3. Infant mortality rates in 1950–1955, 1970–1975, 1985–1990, and projections for the year 2000, and births in 1985–1990, by subregions and countries listed according to mortality level.

Subregion and country	Mortality rate (per 1,000)			Five-yearly decrease		Rate year 2000	Births 1985–1990 (1,000s)
	1950–1955	1970–1975	1985–1990	1950–1970	1970–1985		
Latin America	127	82	55	11.2	8.9	41	12 077
Bolivia	176	151	110	6.1	13.8	69	293
Haiti	220	135	97	21.2	12.8	72	213
Peru	159	110	88	12.1	7.4	63	721
Total							1227
Honduras	196	101	68	23.8	10.7	49	189
Nicaragua	167	100	67	16.8	11.0	42	149
Dominican Republic	149	94	65	14.0	9.5	46	213
Total							551
Brazil	135	91	63	11.1	9.1	48	4086
Ecuador	140	95	63	11.1	10.5	49	328
El Salvador	151	99	60	13.0	13.0	36	182
Guatemala	140	95	59	11.4	12.1	37	350
Total							4946
Paraguay	73	55	49	4.7	2.0	44	139
Mexico	114	71	43	10.7	9.4	28	2438
Colombia	123	73	40	12.5	11.1	33	861
Venezuela	106	49	36	14.4	4.2	30	569
Total							4007
Uruguay	57	46	24	2.8	7.3	16	54
Panama	93	43	23	12.6	6.7	19	61
Argentina	66	49	22	4.2	9.0	17	669
Chile	126	70	18	14.1	17.3	15	301
Costa Rica	94	52	17	10.3	12.5	11	80
Cuba	81	38	13	10.5	7.7	10	181
Total							1346
Non-Latin Caribbean	83	40	21	10.8	6.3	15	146
Guyana	93	56	30	9.2	8.7	21	25
Suriname	89	49	30	10.0	6.3	21	10
Total							35
Trinidad and Tobago	79	30	20	12.2	3.3	14	30
Jamaica	85	36	18	12.2	6.0	14	63
Martinique	65	35	13	7.5	7.3	10	6
Guadeloupe	68	42	12	6.5	10.0	8	7
Barbados	61[a]	27	11	—	-7.3	8	5
Total							111
North America	29	18	10	2.8	2.7	7	4052
United States of America	28	18	10	2.5	2.7	7	3687
Canada	36	16	7	5.0	2.3	7	365

[a] 1955–1960.

Source: CELADE, 1989, and United Nations, 1989.

113

Table 4. Total fertility rate, by subregion and country, 1950–1955 and 1980–2000.

Subregion and country	1950–1955	1980–1985	1985–1990	1990–1995	1995–2000
Latin America	5.9	4.0	3.6	3.3	3.1
Argentina	3.2	3.2	3.0	2.8	2.7
Bolivia	6.8	6.3	6.1	5.8	5.5
Brazil	6.2	3.8	3.5	3.2	2.9
Chile	5.1	2.8	2.7	2.7	2.6
Colombia	6.8	3.5	3.1	2.9	2.8
Costa Rica	6.7	3.5	3.3	3.0	2.8
Cuba	4.1	1.9	1.8	1.9	2.0
Dominican Republic	7.4	4.2	3.8	3.3	3.0
Ecuador	6.9	4.8	4.3	3.9	3.5
El Salvador	6.5	5.2	4.9	4.5	4.2
Guatemala	7.1	6.1	5.8	5.4	4.9
Haiti	6.2	5.1	4.7	4.4	4.1
Honduras	7.1	6.2	5.6	4.9	4.3
Mexico	6.8	4.2	3.6	3.1	2.8
Nicaragua	7.3	5.9	5.5	5.0	4.5
Panama	5.7	3.5	3.1	2.9	2.7
Paraguay	6.8	4.8	4.6	4.3	4.1
Peru	6.9	5.0	4.5	4.0	3.5
Uruguay	2.7	2.6	2.4	2.3	2.3
Venezuela	6.5	4.1	3.8	3.5	3.2
Caribbean[a]	5.2	3.1	2.9	2.8	2.6
Barbados	4.7	1.9	2.0	2.0	2.1
Guadeloupe	5.6	2.6	2.2	2.1	2.1
Jamaica	4.2	3.4	2.9	2.5	2.2
Martinique	5.7	2.1	2.1	2.1	2.1
Puerto Rico	5.0	2.6	2.4	2.3	2.2
Trinidad and Tobago	5.3	2.9	2.7	2.5	2.3
North America[b]	3.5	1.8	1.8	1.8	1.9
Canada	3.7	1.7	1.7	1.7	1.7
United States of America	3.5	1.8	1.8	1.9	1.9

[a] Includes Anguilla, Antigua and Barbuda, Bahamas, Cayman Islands, Dominica, Grenada, Monserrat, Netherlands Antilles, St. Kitts and Nevis, Saint Lucia, St. Vincent and the Grenadines, Turks and Caicos Islands, Virgin Islands (UK), and Virgin Islands (USA).

[b] Includes Bermuda, Greenland, and Saint Pierre and Miguelón.

Source: CELADE, 1990, and United Nations, 1989.

Table 5. Coverage of drinking water supply and sanitation in 25 countries of the Americas, up to December 1988 (population in thousands).

Country	Total population	Urban population	Rural population	Drinking water supply — Total population served: With connection	With easy access	Total	% of country's population	Drinking water supply — Urban population served: With connection	With easy access	Total	% of urban population	Drinking water supply — Rural population served: Total	% of rural population
Argentina	31 074	26 219	4855	18 208	1763	19 971	64.27	18 208	944	19 152	73.05	819	16.87
Bahamas	241	136	105	126	114	240	99.59	126	9	135	99.26	105	100.00
Barbados	253	89	164	87	165	252	99.60	87	2	89	100.00	163	99.39
Belize	175	90	85	70	65	135	77.14	70	5	75	83.33	60	70.59
Bolivia	6928	3471	3457	2311	898	3209	46.32	2311	374	2685	77.36	524	15.16
Brazil	144 426	106 587	37 839	96 577	42 252	138 829	96.12	96 577	9832	106 409	99.83	32 420	85.68
Chile	12 748	10 497	2251	10 287	672	10 959	85.97	10 287	210	10 497	100.00	462	20.52
Colombia	31 200	22 100	9100	14 500	12 800	27 300	87.50	14 500	4900	19 400	87.78	7900	86.81
Costa Rica	2866	1719	1147	1685	997	2682	93.58	1685	34	1719	100.00	963	83.96
Dominican Republic	6866	4038	2828	1913	1624	3537	51.51	1913	820	2733	67.68	804	28.43
Ecuador	10 203	5529	4674	3963	1918	5881	57.64	3963	190	4153	75.11	1728	36.97
El Salvador	5032	2349	2683	1672	379	2051	40.76	1672	110	1782	75.86	269	10.03
Guatemala	8681	3287	5394	2393	2830	5223	60.17	2393	608	3001	91.30	2222	41.19
Guyana	756	246	510	196	413	609	80.56	196	34	230	93.50	379	74.31
Haiti	5562	1581	3981	474	1851	2325	41.80	474	403	877	55.47	1448	36.37
Honduras	4625	1947	2678	1600	1747	3347	72.37	1600	140	1740	89.37	1607	60.01
Mexico	89 500	63 500	26 000	47 000	14 498	61 498	68.71	47 000	3928	50 928	80.20	10 570	40.65
Nicaragua	3622	2109	1513	1436	492	1928	53.23	1436	206	1642	77.86	286	18.90
Panama	2282	1111	1171	1063	823	1886	82.65	1063	48	1111	100.00	775	66.18
Paraguay	3900	1733	2167	866	420	1286	32.97	866	260	1126	64.97	160	7.38
Peru	21 256	13 890	7366	8679	3743	12 422	58.44	8679	2100	10 779	77.60	1643	22.31
Suriname	395	296	99	2	282	284	71.90	2	229	231	78.04	53	53.54
Trinidad and Tobago	1230	840	390	730	450	1180	95.93	730	110	840	100.00	340	87.18
Uruguay	2990	2607	384	2387	152	2539	84.92	2387	132	2519	96.62	20	5.21
Venezuela	18 757	15 604	3153	12 142	4614	16 756	89.33	12 142	1814	13 956	89.44	2800	88.80
Total	415 568	291 575	123 994	230 367	95 962	326 329	78.53	230 367	27 442	257 809	88.42	68 520	55.26

115

Table 5 (cont.). Coverage of drinking water supply and sanitation in 25 countries of the Americas up to December 1988 (population in thousands).

Sewerage and excreta disposal

Country	Total population served				Urban population served				Rural population served	
	With connection	Other	Total	% of country's population	With connection	Other	Total	% of urban population	Total	% of rural population
Argentina	10 261	17 379	27 640	88.95	10 261	15 958	26 219	100.00	1421	29.27
Bahamas	22a	114a	136a	56.43a	22	114	136	100.00	0a	0.00a
Barbados	18a	24a	42a	16.60a	18	24	42	47.19	0a	0.00a
Belize	20	107	127	72.57	20	55	75	83.33	52	61.18
Bolivia	1394	960	2354	33.98	1394	520	1914	55.14	440	12.73
Brazil	45 000	68 155	113 155	78.35	45 000	49 896	94 896	89.03	18 259	48.25
Chile	8654	1983	10 637	83.44	8654	1843	10 497	100.00	140	6.22
Colombia	12 000	8300	20 300	65.06	12 000	6700	18 700	84.62	1600	17.58
Costa Rica	722	2063	2785	97.17	722	997	1719	100.00	1066	92.94
Dominican Republic	882	3220	4102	59.74	882	2209	3091	76.55	1011	35.75
Ecuador	3441	2317	5758	56.43	3441	719	4160	75.24	1598	34.19
El Salvador	1339	1706	3045	60.51	1339	671	2010	85.57	1035	38.58
Guatemala	1617	3325	4942	56.93	1617	741	2358	71.74	2584	47.91
Guyana	70	577	647	85.58	70	138	208	84.55	439	86.08
Haiti	0	1228	1228	22.08	0	650	650	41.11	578	14.52
Honduras	1178	1709	2887	62.42	1178	539	1717	88.19	1170	43.69
Mexico	33 518	6917	40 435	45.18	33 518	4689	38 207	60.17	2228	8.57
Nicaragua	685a	0a	685a	18.91a	685	:::	685a	32.48a	0a	0.00a
Panama	805	1104	1909	83.65	805	305	1110	99.91	799	68.23
Paraguay	437	1810	2247	57.62	437	510	947	54.65	1300	59.99
Peru	7640	1223a	8863a	41.70a	7640	:::	7640a	55.00a	1223	16.60
Suriname	9	212	221	55.95	9	178	187	63.18	34	34.34
Trinidad and Tobago	250	970	1220	99.19	250	590	840	100.00	380	97.44
Uruguay	1436	370	1806	60.40	1436	119	1555	59.65	251	65.36
Venezuela	10 611	6719	17 330	92.39	10 611	4509	15 120	96.90	2210	70.09
Total	142 009	132 492	274 501	66.05	142 009	92 674	234 683	80.49	39 818	32.11

aInsufficient data.

116

Table 6. Vaccine coverage in the Region of the Americas, 1989–1990.

Subregion and country	Population (less than 1 year)		OPV3 %		DPT3 %		Measles %		BCG %	
	89	90	89	90	89	90	89	90	89	90
Andean Subregion	2 456 562	2 363 278	69	76	60	71	55	67	72	79
Bolivia	261 582	221 956	49	50	39	41	47	53	28	48
Colombia	669 809	685 108	90	93	78	87	64	82	94	95
Ecuador	316 622	320 852	64	67	55	68	57	61	91	88
Peru	670 000	600 904	60	73	58	72	52	64	62	83
Venezuela	538 549	534 458	67	72	55	63	50	62	68	63
Brazil[a]	4 307 582	3 610 961	97	93	54	81	58	78	70	78
Central America	989 404	1 016 513	71	80	65	74	69	78	59	70
Belize	6701	7200	71	80	71	84	68	81	87	80
Costa Rica	82 451	82 500	87	95	87	95	78	90	90	92
El Salvador	182 173	186 267	64	76	64	76	73	75	63	60
Guatemala	339 385	349 847	58	74	50	66	54	68	21	62
Honduras	174 262	180 721	86	87	85	84	94	90	80	71
Nicaragua	143 200	148 085	85	86	66	65	63	82	92	81
Panama	61 232	61 893	72	86	70	86	73	99	87	97
Southern Cone	1 144 876	1 090 660	83	90	82	88	85	92	88	98
Argentina	677 398	602 288	86	89	80	85	89	95	92	99
Chile	279 150	293 556	95	99	95	99	91	98	95	97
Paraguay[a]	134 928	138 802	41	76	61	78	53	69	53	90
Uruguay	53 400	56 014	88	88	88	88	82	82	99	99
Latin Caribbean	606 619	616 560	71	74	61	67	56	73	57	79
Cuba[a]	187 529	186 658	95	94	95	92	97	94	97	98
Haiti	201 707	207 637	50	40	50	41	31	31	40	72
Dominican Republic[a]	217 383	222 265	70	90	43	69	43	96	38	68
Mexico	2 579 200	1 970 515	96	96	65	66	85	78	80	70
Latin America	12 084 243	10 668 487	86	87	62	75	66	77	73	78
English-speaking										
Caribbean	131 672	134 637	82	86	82	86	72	75	61	62
Anguilla	157	200	99	99	99	99	92	99	99	99
Antigua and Barbuda	1088	1114	99	99	99	99	95	89	–	–
Bahamas	5641	6013	82	82	86	86	87	87	–	–
Barbados	4032	4040	80	90	78	91	85	87	–	–
Cayman Islands	378	434	93	99	93	99	89	89	81	81
Dominica	1715	1745	94	94	92	94	88	88	99	99
Grenada	2613	2650	86	69	87	80	89	85	–	–
Guyana	17 658	18 500	79	79	77	83	69	73	76	85
Jamaica	57 487	59 104	84	87	85	86	71	74	99	98
Montserrat	199	154	93	99	93	99	89	99	60	99
Saint Kitts and Nevis	924	980	99	99	99	99	90	99	...	...
Saint Lucia	3530	4380	93	90	92	89	91	82	99	94
Saint Vincent and the Grenadines	2482	2505	97	92	98	98	99	96	99	99
Suriname	10 000	9000	71	81	72	83	73	65	–	–
Trinidad and Tobago	23 280	23 280	77	87	77	82	59	70	–	–
Turks and Caicos Islands	250	300	89	98	89	97	76	81	99	99
British Virgin Islands	238	238	97	99	99	99	87	99	99	99
North America	3 998 895	4 009 883	...	...	...	...	...	...	...	...
Bermuda	895	883	76	62	74	62	67	63	–	–
Canada	358 000	362 000	...	...	...	...	...	...	...	...
USA	3 640 000	3 647 000	...	...	...	...	...	...	...	...
Total[b]	16 214 810	14 813 007	86	87	62	76	66	77	73	78

[a]Coverage calculated with two doses of OPV.
[b]Total coverage does not include North America.
– Vaccine not in use.
... No data available.
Source: PAHO (provisional data).

117

Table 7. Some primary health care indicators reported.

Country or other political unit	Infant mortality rate		Life expectancy at birth			Maternal mortality rate (per 10,000 live births)		% Newborns with weight under 2,500 g	
	Year	Value	Year	M	F	Year	Value	Year	Value
Anguilla	1988	38	1988	71.0	74.0		w/i	1988	6.9
Antigua and Barbuda	1990	20	1990	—72.0—			w/i	1990	5.2
Argentina	1989	23	1985–1990	70.6	74.0	1987	4.9	w/i	w/i
Bahamas	1988	21	w/i	w/i	w/i	1988–1989	3.7	1989	7.8
Barbados	1988	19	1988	70.2	75.2		w/i	1988	16.0
Belize	1989	19	1990	69.9	71.8	1989	3.6	1989	2.7
Bolivia	1979–1989	96		w/i	w/i	1988	24.7	1988	9.3
Brazil	1987	51		w/i	w/i		w/i	1989	11.5
British Virgin Islands	1990	9	1990	67.2	75.6	1990	0	1990	8.0
Canada	1988	7	1985–1987	73.0	79.7	1988	0.5	1988	6.0
Cayman Islands	1990	7	1990	—74.5—		1990	0.8	1990	8.7
Chile	1989	17	1985–1990	—71.5—		w/i	4.1	1989	7.1
Colombia	1989	38	1989	65.9	71.7	1989	4.0	1988	12.8
Costa Rica	1989	14	1985–1990	—74.7—		1989	3.0	w/i	6.2
Cuba	1990	11	1985–1990	73.5	77.1	1989	2.9	1989	7.3
Dominica	1988	18	1990	—76.0—		1990	0.0	1988	10.0
Dominican Republic	1990	65	1985–1990	63.9	68.1	1990	9.0	1989	13.7
Ecuador	1988	45	1985–1990	63.4	67.6	1988	15.6		w/i
El Salvador	1986	58	1985–1990	58.0	66.0	1989	12.7	w/i	w/i
Guatemala	w/i	w/i	w/i	w/i	w/i		w/i		9.2
Grenada	1988	24	1990	—71.5—			w/i	1988	12.0
Guyana	1986	49	w/i	65.8	70.8		w/i	1986	10
Haiti	1988	103	w/i	54.9	58.4	1989	23.0	w/i	8.7
Honduras	1988	56	w/i	w/i	w/i	1990	22.1	1988	11.1
Jamaica	w/i	w/i	1989	—70.8—			w/i	1988	5.0
Mexico	1987	31	1990	66.3	72.7	1987	5.6	1989	9.2
Montserrat	1988	24	1988	63.5	69.8		w/i	1988	12.0
Nicaragua	1990	72	1985–1990	—63.3—		w/i	w/i	1986	8.1
Panama	1988	23	w/i	70.4	74.5	w/i	6.0	w/i	5.2
Paraguay	1990	47	1990	65.2	69.5	1990	27.0	1990	7.5
Peru	1989	88	1989	—62.7—		1989	24.0	w/i	11.3
Saint Kitts and Nevis	w/i	w/i	1988	—67.0—			w/i	1988	9.0
Saint Lucia	1988	15	1988	67.9	73.7	1988	0	1988	1.0
Saint Vincent and the Grenadines	1988	22					0.6		w/i
Suriname	1990	25	1990	66.9	72.2	1990	3.1	1988	w/i
Trinidad and Tobago	1988	15	1990	w/i	w/i	1987	5.4		w/i
United States	1989	10	1985–1990	—71.6—		1987	0.7		w/i
Uruguay	1988	21	1985–1990	67.8	74.4	1989	2.5		7.6
Venezuela	1988	23	1988	70.0	75.4	1988	6.0	1986	w/i

118

Table 8. Demographic indicators reported.

Country or other political unit	Population			Crude death rate		Crude birth rate		Total fertility rate		% Women using contraceptives	
	Year	Number in thousands	% rural	Year	Value	Year	Value	Year	Value	Year	Value
Anguilla	1988	7	w/i		w/i		w/i		w/i		w/i
Antigua and Barbuda	1988	79	w/i								
Argentina	1990	w/i	14	1985–1990	8.6	1985–1990	21.4	1985–1990	w/i		w/i
Bahamas	1990	254	w/i	1988	5.4	1988	20.2		w/i		w/i
Barbados	1991	257	10		w/i		w/i	1985–1990	1.8	1990	w/i
Belize	1990	184	13		w/i		w/i	1989	5.2	1989	10
Bolivia	1988	6400	49		w/i		w/i	1989	5.0	1990	12
Brazil	1988	144 400	26		w/i		w/i		w/i	1986	43
British Virgin Islands	1991	12	72		w/i		w/i		w/i		w/i
Canada	1990	26 600	w/i		w/i		w/i		w/i		w/i
Cayman Islands	1991	27	w/i		w/i		w/i	1985–1990	3.4		w/i
Chile	1990	13 200	18	1989	5.8	1989	23.4		w/i		w/i
Colombia	1989	32 300	35	1985–1990	6.1	1989–1990	27.4	1990	3.1	1990	40
Costa Rica	1990	3015	54	1989	3.8	1989	28.5		w/i		w/i
Cuba	1989	10 500	27	1989	6.4	1989	17.6		w/i	1987	78
Dominica	1991	81	67		w/i		w/i		w/i	1988	54
Dominican Republic	w/i	w/i	w/i	1985–1990	6.8	1985–1990	31.3	1985–1990	3.6		w/i
Ecuador	1988	10 200	w/i		w/i		w/i		w/i	1988	32
El Salvador	1991	5400	57		w/i	1990	36.3	1990	4.5	w/i	w/i
Guatemala	w/i	w/i	w/i		w/i		w/i		w/i		w/i
Grenada	1988	108	w/i		w/i		w/i	1985–1990	3.5	1990	54
Guyana	w/i	w/i	w/i		w/i		w/i		w/i		w/i
Haiti	1989	5750	85	1989	13	1989	36	1989	5.7	1988	11
Honduras	1989	4950	w/i		w/i	1987	38.0		w/i	1989	2
Jamaica	w/i	w/i	w/i		w/i		w/i		w/i		w/i
Mexico	1990	81 150	33	1987	5.0	1987	34	1986	3.8	w/i	w/i
Montserrat	1991	12	w/i		w/i		w/i	1985–1990	2.3	1985	50
Nicaragua	1990	3871	43	1985–1990	7.9	1985–1990	42		w/i		w/i
Panama	1990	2400	47		w/i		w/i		w/i	1990	58
Paraguay	1991	4397	58		w/i		w/i		w/i	1990	44
Peru	1989	21 500	w/i	1989	9.4	1990	32.9		w/i	1985–1990	8
Saint Kitts and Nevis	1991	44	w/i		w/i		w/i	1985–1990	3.0	1988	41
Saint Lucia	1991	148	w/i		w/i		w/i	1985–1990	3.6	1985	43
Saint Vincent and the Grenadines	1991	114	51		w/i		w/i	1985–1990	3.8	1990	61
Suriname	w/i	400	10		w/i		w/i		w/i	1990	55
Trinidad and Tobago	1990	1300	30		6.1		w/i	1990	2.8	1987	53
United States	w/i	w/i	w/i		w/i	1988	15.9	1988	3.8	1988	60
Uruguay	1989	3050	w/i		w/i	1989	18.1		w/i	w/i	w/i
Venezuela	1989	19 250	16	1988	4.4	1989	27.5	1989	3.3	1989	14

w/i: without information.

119

Table 9. Coverage and resources (reported data).

Country or other political unit	Pregnant women attended %						Infant delivery %		Physicians		Nursing personnel		Hospital beds	
	With tet-tox		During pregnancy		During delivery									
	Year	Value	Year	Value	Year	Value	Year	Value	Year	Number	Year	Number	Year	Number
Anguilla		w/i	1990	100	1990	100	1990	100		w/i		w/i	w/i	w/i
Antigua and Barbuda		w/i	1990	100	1990	100	1990	100		w/i		w/i		w/i
Argentina		w/i	1988	96	1987	95	1990	100	1985	90 000	1988	64 000	1985	147 000
Bahamas	1989	62	1989	99	1989	99		w/i	1990	330	1990	630(x)	1990	1100
Barbados		w/i	1990	100	1990	100	1990	100		w/i		w/i		w/i
Belize	1989	39	1989	92	1989	83	1989	95	1990	120	1990	300	1990	390
Bolivia	1990	60	1989	38	1989	29	1989	29	1989	3700	1989	4000(x)	1991	9500
Brazil	1990	63	1988	65		w/i		w/i	1988	170 000	1988	161 000	1987	500 000
British Virgin Islands		w/i						w/i		w/i		w/i		w/i
Canada		w/i	1990	100	1990	100	1990	100	1988	57 400	1988	269 000	1989	183 000
Cayman Islands	1990	95	1988	89	1988	100	1988	100		w/i		w/i		w/i
Chile		w/i		w/i	1989	99	1988	81	1990	14 200		w/i	1989	40 900
Colombia	1989	27	1989	59	1989	59	1989	100	1989	29 700		w/i	1989	42 900
Costa Rica	1990	7	1989	91	1989	94	1986	91	1991	3100	1991	8400		w/i
Cuba	1989	95	1989	100	1989	100	1989	100	1990	39 000	1990	65 000	1990	57 600
Dominica		w/i	1990	100	1990	100	1990	100		w/i		w/i		w/i
Dominican Republic		w/i	1990	43	1990	44	1990	w/i		w/i		w/i		w/i
Ecuador		w/i	1988	47	1988	26	1990	65	1988	10 900	1988	15 300	w/i	w/i
El Salvador	1990	40		w/i		w/i	1988	w/i		w/i		w/i		w/i
Guatemala	w/i	12	1988	34	1988	23		w/i		w/i		w/i	1989	7500(x)
Haiti	1989	75	1988	43	w/i	20	w/i	89		943	1989	200		w/i
Grenada		w/i	1990	100	1990	100	1990	100		w/i		w/i		w/i
Guyana	w/i	47	w/i	95	w/i	98	w/i	98		w/i		w/i		w/i
Honduras	1989	20	1989	77	1989	63	1990	70		w/i		w/i	1990	4000(x)
Jamaica		w/i	1990	67	1989	79	1989	68		w/i		w/i	1989	5700(x)
Mexico	1989	39	1989	50	1989	45	1989	97	1990	85 000(x)	1990	29 000(x)	1990	49 000(x)
Nicaragua		w/i	1990	87	1989	42	1989	100		w/i		w/i		w/i
Montserrat		w/i	1990	100	1990	100	1990	80		w/i		w/i		w/i
Panama		w/i	1990	82	1990	85	1990	64	1989	2800	1989	5900	1989	5400
Paraguay	1990	69	1990	60	1990	60	1990	w/i	1990	3000	1990	3000	1990	32 400
Peru	1990	3		w/i		w/i	1990	w/i	1990	23 000	1990	18 000		w/i
Saint Kitts and Nevis		S/I	1990	100	1990	100	1990	100		w/i	1989	w/i		w/i
Saint Lucia		w/i	1990	100	1990	100	1990	100		w/i		w/i		w/i
Saint Vincent and the Grenadines							1990	100						
Suriname		w/i	1990	100	1989	90		w/i	1989	320	1989	1340	1990	1900
Trinidad and Tobago	w/i	w/i	1988	98	1989	w/i	w/i	w/i		w/i		w/i	1990	w/i
United States of America	1989	85	1988	98	1988	99	1988	100	1989	600 000	1989	1 600 000		w/i
Uruguay		w/i		w/i	1989	100		w/i		w/i		w/i		w/i
Venezuela		w/i		w/i	1989	82		w/i	1988	30 500	1988	54 400	1990	51 600

(x) Only public sector.
w/i: without information.

120

Table 10. Selected socioeconomic indicators.

Country or other political unit	GNP per capita 1990	GDP per capita growth 1988-1990	External debt as % of GNP 1989	Consumer price index 1990	Illiteracy 15 years and + 1990 T	M	F	% Central gvmt. expend. on health 1989	Human development index 1990	Aver. annual growth rate gross domestic investment (%) 1980-1989
Anguilla	w/i	w/i	w/i	w/i	w/i	w/i	w/i	w/i	w/i	w/i
Antigua and Barbuda	3690	w/i	w/i	w/i	w/i	w/i	w/i	w/i	0.832	w/i
Argentina	2260	-9.1	94	1853	4.7	4.5	4.9	2.0	0.854	-7.8
Bahamas	11 370(1)	+9.8	n/a	6(1)	4.8	5.2	4.4	w/i	w/i	w/i
Barbados	6370(1)	7.5	w/i	w/i	2	2	2	w/i	0.945	w/i
Belize	1720(1)	24.2(2)	42	w/i	5	w/i	w/i	w/i	0.700	w/i
Bolivia	620(1)	8.4	99	18	22.5	15.3	29.5	6.6	0.416	-11.6
Brazil	2340(1)	0.0	39	2360	22.2	20.9	23.4	6.1	0.759	0.7
Canada	19 020(1)	25.0(2)	n/a	5(1)	w/i	w/i	w/i	5.5	0.983	5.6
Chile	1890	20.0	79	29	6.6	6.5	6.8	5.9	0.878	2.7
Colombia	1200	11.0	44	31	13.3	12.5	14.1	w/i	0.757	0.3
Costa Rica	1940	12.8	92	22	7.2	7.4	6.9	27.2	0.876	4.9
Cuba	w/i	w/i	w/i	w/i	6.0	5.0	7.0	w/i	0.754	w/i
Dominica	1680	w/i	w/i	w/i	6	6	6	w/i	0.800	w/i
Dominican Republic	790(1)	5.3(2)	74	45	20.0	18.0	21.4	w/i	0.622	5.4
Ecuador	1010	16.8	107	48	14.2	12.2	16.2	9.8	0.655	-3.2
El Salvador	1090	5.7	34	20	27.0	23.8	30.0	7.4	0.524	2.7
Guatemala	910	11.2	32	50	44.9	36.9	52.9	w/i	0.488	-2.4
Haiti	360(1)	-1.7	35	13	47.0	40.9	52.6	w/i	0.296	-3.8
Grenada	1900(1)	72.0(2)	w/i	w/i	4	2	6	w/i	0.751	w/i
Guyana	340	-9.4	63	w/i	3.6	2.5	4.6	w/i	0.589	-0.5
Honduras	900(1)	-6.2	75	25	26.9	24.5	29.4	w/i	0.492	3.7
Jamaica	1260(1)	9.6	143	17(1)	1.6	1.8	1.4	w/i	0.761	w/i
Cayman Islands	w/i	w/i	w/i	w/i	2.0	w/i	w/i	w/i	w/i	w/i
British Virgin Islands	w/i	w/i	w/i	w/i	w/i	w/i	w/i	w/i	w/i	w/i
Mexico	w/i	6.9	60	30	12.7	10.5	14.9	1.7	0.838	-5.0
Nicaragua	w/i	-22.3	w/i	8500	20	w/i	w/i	w/i	0.612	w/i
Montserrat	w/i	w/i	w/i	w/i	w/i	w/i	w/i	w/i	w/i	w/i
Panama	1830	-15.8	139	1	11.9	11.9	11.8	19.8	0.796	-15.6
Paraguay	1150	6.7	58	43	10	8	12	w/i	0.667	w/i
Peru	1090	-22.1	93	8300	14.9	8.5	21.3	5.5	0.644	-4.5
Saint Kitts and Nevis	1810(1)	w/i	w/i	w/i	10	10	10	w/i	w/i	w/i
Saint Lucia	w/i	w/i	w/i	w/i	18	18	18	w/i	0.699	w/i
Saint Vincent and the Grenadines	1360(1)	w/i	w/i	w/i	w/i	w/i	w/i	w/i	0.636	w/i
Suriname	3020(1)	w/i	n/a	w/i	5.1	4.9	5.3	w/i	0.792	w/i
Trinidad and Tobago	3230(1)	-7.0	49	11	5.1	3.5	6.6	w/i	0.876	7.7
United States of America	21 000(1)	13.1(2)	n/a	5(1)	0.5	w/i	w/i	12.9	0.976	4.7
Uruguay	2620(1)	2.0	47	130	3.8	3.4	4.1	4.5	0.905	-7.9
Venezuela	2420	3.0	70	32	11.9	13.3	10.4	w/i	0.848	-3.8

(1) 1989
(2) 1988–1989
n/a: not applicable
w/i: without information
Sources: a) GNP, external debt, gross domestic investment: ECLAC, World Bank. b) GDP per capita growth, CPI: ECLAC, World Bank. c) Illiteracy: UNESCO. d) Human Development Index: UNDP.
e) Central Government Expenditure on Health: IMF.

121

Index

Main references are in bold type.

INDEX